BASIC DRUG
CALCULATIONS

BASIC DRUG CALCULATIONS

Meta Brown, R.N., M.A.

Director, Division of Nursing,
Maricopa Technical Community College,
Phoenix, Arizona

Joyce L. Mulholland, R.N.C., M.A., M.S.

Professor, Division of Nursing,
Maricopa Technical Community College,
Phoenix, Arizona

Second edition

THE C. V. MOSBY COMPANY

ST. LOUIS   TORONTO   1984

MOSBY

A TRADITION OF PUBLISHING EXCELLENCE

Editor: Julie Cardamon
Assistant editor: Bess Arends
Manuscript editor: Carlotta Seely
Book design: Gail Morey Hudson
Cover design: Suzanne Oberholtzer
Production: Carolyn Biby, Teresa Breckwoldt, Ginny Douglas

SECOND EDITION

The C.V. Mosby Company
11830 Westline Industrial Drive, St. Louis, Missouri 63146

Library of Congress Cataloging in Publication Data

Brown, Meta.
  Basic drug calculations.

  1.   Pharmaceutical arithmetic—Problems, exercises, etc.
I.   Mulholland, Joyce L.   II.   Title.
RS57.B76   1984   615'.4'01513   83-13462
ISBN 0-8016-0863-5

AC/VH/VH 9 8 7 6 5 4 3   03/D/374

Preface

The purpose of this workbook is to help the health professional understand basic metrology. Experience has proved that the use of realistic problems and immediate feedback are the most effective educational methods.

This book is divided into 11 sections. Each section is made up of units that present specific objectives. In order to obtain the full benefit from this workbook, the student should review Appendix A, Abbreviations for Medications, before beginning Section 1. The material is correlated in a sequential process starting with basic mathematics; therefore it is important to proceed in an orderly fashion. All answers are worked out completely and are adjacent to the worksheet for immediate verification of process and answers. After completing all worksheets and verifying the answers, the student should take the quiz at the end of the section. Students who have demonstrated competence in all phases of general mathematics may wish to begin with the general math quiz at the end of Section 1. Since a strong foundation in mathematics is *essential* for success, most students will benefit from a thorough study of all of the General Mathematics units. When all sections have been completed, the student should take the comprehensive quiz that follows Section 11.

The ratio and proportion method is used throughout the book. It has been our experience that this mode of problem solving contributes to the greatest long-term understanding and retention of the mathematics process. The ratio and proportion method also has a built-in, easy means of proving each problem to ensure correct calculation of medication.

The Children's Dosages section reflects the most common methods of calculating safe dosages. The revised Insulin and Heparin sections present the most essential information for current practice. The Intravenous Calculations section now contains basic titration calculations pertaining to milligrams per kilogram in 24 hours, milligrams per minute, and units per milliliter.

The basic objectives for this book can be divided in the following way:

Basic math objectives

Given basic mathematical problems, the student will solve the following types of problems:
1. Fractions
2. Decimals
3. Conversion of fractions to decimals
4. Conversion of decimals to fractions
5. Multiplication of numbers by 10, 100, 1000

6. Division of numbers by 10, 100, 1000
7. Percentages

Given a basic ratio and proportion problem, the student will:
1. Set up the problem correctly.
2. Identify one- and two-step problems.

Basic metric and apothecary objectives

Given basic metric and apothecary problems, the student will:
1. Solve basic math problems encountered in daily hospital practice.
2. Convert the metric system to the apothecary system using ratio and proportion.
3. Convert the apothecary system to the metric system using ratio and proportion.
4. Solve intravenous-solution computations involving drops per minute and milliliters per hour, milligrams per kilogram, milligrams per minutes, and units per milliliter.
5. Solve basic solution problems.
6. Prepare medications from powder or crystals.
7. Convert insulin units to milliliters.
8. Convert heparin units to milliliters.
9. Calculate safe children's dosages.
10. Estimate answers before working problems.
11. Validate answers.

We sincerely hope that this workbook will serve as a source of basic practical information. The instructor will act as a reference person, since the book is self-explanatory.

We are very grateful to Betty Gahart, R.N., author of *Intravenous Medications,* for allowing us to quote safe ranges of intravenous medications and to the publishers of *Physicians' Desk Reference* for giving us permission to quote medication dosage ranges.

In addition, we especially appreciate the efforts of Helen Jackson, who spent many hours typing the manuscript.

Meta Brown
Joyce Mulholland

Guide for students

This book contains 11 sections and a comprehensive quiz. Each section consists of units. Start with Section 1, which is General Mathematics. Examples and explanations are given on the first page of each unit. After you have completed all the worksheets in Section 1, Units A to P, take the general math quiz at the end of the section. If you do not get 100%, review the unit containing those items missed. Do not proceed to Section 2 unless you understand all the units in Section 1 thoroughly.

Section 2 is Ratio and Proportion. Start with Unit A and complete all units. Take the quiz after the completion of all units in Section 2. Do not proceed to Section 3 unless you thoroughly understand all units in Section 2 and obtain 100% on the quiz.

Proceed through the remainder of the sections in the same manner as stated above.

REMEMBER: Medical personnel are accountable for their actions. The patient's rights must be respected. Below are five patient's rights that must be strictly followed for maximum patient safety:
1. Right medication
2. Right dosage
3. Right time
4. Right route
5. Right patient

There are quizzes for the following sections only. Answer sheets are placed immediately after each quiz.

Section 1   General mathematics
Section 2   Ratio and proportion
Section 3   Metric system
Section 4   Apothecary system
Section 5   Apothecary-metric conversions
Section 6   Intravenous calculations: drop factors and basic titrations
Section 9   Insulin
Section 11   Children's dosages

Comprehensive quiz

Contents

General mathematics

UNIT A

Math objectives

1. *Convert fractions into whole numbers.*
2. *Convert fractions into mixed numbers.*
3. *Reduce fractions to lowest terms.*

A fraction is part of a whole number. The fraction $^6/_8$ means that there are 8 parts to the whole number (bottom) but you want to measure only 6 of those parts (top number).

$^6/_8$ can be reduced by division of both the numbers by 2.

$$\frac{6 \div 2}{8 \div 2} = \frac{3}{4}$$

Changing improper fractions into whole or mixed numbers

An improper fraction has a large top number and a small bottom number, such as $^8/_4$.

RULE:
1 When the top number is larger than the bottom number, divide the bottom number into the top number.
2 Write the remainder as a fraction and reduce to lowest terms.

EXAMPLE:

$^8/_4 = 8 \div 4 = 2$ *Whole number*

$^{16}/_6 = 16 \div 6 = 2^4/_6 = 2^2/_3$ *This is a mixed number* because it has a whole number plus a fraction.

Section 1 answer sheets begin on p. 24.

1A Worksheet

Change the following to whole numbers or mixed fractions:

1. $\frac{8}{8}$ =

2. $\frac{13}{4}$ =

3. $\frac{6}{2}$ =

4. $\frac{14}{9}$ =

5. $\frac{34}{6}$ =

6. $\frac{100}{25}$ =

7. $\frac{7}{4}$ =

8. $\frac{120}{64}$ =

9. $\frac{12}{4}$ =

10. $\frac{41}{6}$ =

UNIT B

Math objective

Change mixed numbers into improper fractions.

Changing mixed numbers into improper fractions

RULE:
1 Multiply the whole number by the bottom number of the fraction.
2 Add this to the top number of the fraction.
3 Write the sum as the top number of the fraction; the bottom number of the fraction remains the same.

EXAMPLE:

$$2^3/_8 = \frac{8 \times 2 + 3}{8} = {}^{19}/_8$$

$$4^2/_5 = \frac{20 + 2}{5} = {}^{22}/_5$$

1B Worksheet

Change the following to improper fractions:

1. $1^1/_5 =$

2. $1^1/_4 =$

3. $16^1/_3 =$

4. $3^7/_{12} =$

5. $13^3/_5 =$

6. $4^3/_8 =$

7. $3^5/_6 =$

8. $2^5/_8 =$

9. $10^3/_6 =$

10. $125^2/_3 =$

3

UNIT C

Math objectives

1. *Find lowest common denominators in fractions.*
2. *Add fractions.*
3. *Add mixed numbers.*
4. *Add fractions and mixed numbers and reduce to lowest terms (reduce fractions).*

Addition of fractions and mixed numbers

Finding lowest common bottom number (in fraction)

RULE: **1** Find the lowest common number that the bottom numbers can be divided into.

2 Change the fractions to equivalent fractions using these bottom numbers.

EXAMPLE: $2/3 = {}^{16}/_{24}$

$7/8 = {}^{21}/_{24}$

$1/6 = {}^{4}/_{24}$

Addition of fractions and mixed numbers

RULE: **1** If fractions have the same bottom number, add the top numbers, write over the bottom number, and reduce.

EXAMPLE:
$$\frac{1}{5}$$
$$+\frac{2}{5}$$
$$\overline{\frac{3}{5}}$$

2 If fractions have different bottom numbers, find the lowest common bottom number and then add the top numbers.

EXAMPLE:
$$\frac{3}{5} = \frac{9}{15}$$
$$+\frac{2}{3} = \frac{10}{15}$$
$$\overline{\frac{19}{15}} = 19 \div 15 = 1^4/_{15}$$

3 To add mixed numbers, first add the fractions and then add this to the sum of the whole numbers.

EXAMPLE:
$$9^5/_8 = 9^{15}/_{24}$$
$$+6^1/_6 = 6\ ^4/_{24}$$
$$\overline{\hphantom{+6^1/_6 =\ }15^{19}/_{24}}$$

1C Worksheet

Add the following fractions and mixed numbers:

1. $1/5$
$+2/5$

5. $1/8$
$1/4$
$+2/9$

2. $3/5$
$+2/3$

6. $7/9$
$4/5$
$+9/10$

3. $6^1/6$
$+9^5/8$

7. $3^1/4$
$+9^3/4$

4. $1^3/8$
$+9^9/10$

8. $8^2/5$
$14^7/10$
$+ \ 9^9/10$

UNIT D

Math objectives

1. *Subtract fractions.*
2. *Subtract mixed numbers.*

Subtraction of fractions and mixed numbers

RULE: **1** If fractions have the same bottom number, find the difference between the top numbers and write it over the common number. Reduce the fraction if necessary.

EXAMPLE:

$$\begin{array}{r} {}^{27}/_{32} \\ -{}^{18}/_{32} \\ \hline {}^{9}/_{32} \end{array}$$

Difference between the top numbers (27 minus 18) equals 9. Bottom number is 32.

RULE: **2** If fractions have different bottom numbers, find the lowest common bottom number and proceed as above.

EXAMPLE:

$$\begin{array}{r} {}^{7}/_{8} = {}^{21}/_{24} \\ -{}^{2}/_{3} = {}^{16}/_{24} \\ \hline {}^{5}/_{24} \end{array}$$

Difference between the top numbers (21 minus 16) equals 5. Bottom number is 24.

RULE: **3** To subtract mixed numbers, first subtract the fractions and then find the difference in the whole numbers. If the fraction in the bottom number is larger than the fraction in the top number, you cannot subtract it. You must borrow from the whole number before subtracting the fraction.

EXAMPLE:

$$\begin{array}{r} 21\,{}^{7}/_{16} \\ -\ 7\,{}^{12}/_{16} \end{array}$$

You cannot subtract the top numbers because 12 is larger than 7. Therefore you must make a whole number out of $^{7}/_{16}$ and add the 7.

$$^{16}/_{16} + {}^{7}/_{16} = {}^{23}/_{16}$$

Since we added a whole number to the fraction, we must take a whole number away from 21 and make it 20. The problem now is set up as follows:

$$21^{7}/_{16} = 20^{16}/_{16} + {}^{7}/_{16} = \begin{array}{r} 20^{23}/_{16} \\ -\ 7^{12}/_{16} \\ \hline 13^{11}/_{16} \end{array}$$

RULE: **4** Reduce answer to lowest terms.

1D Worksheet

Subtract fractions and mixed numbers (reduce answer to lowest terms):

1. $\begin{array}{r} {}^4/_5 \\ -\,{}^1/_2 \\ \hline \end{array}$

2. $\begin{array}{r} 7\,{}^{16}/_{24} \\ -\,3\,{}^1/_8 \\ \hline \end{array}$

3. $\begin{array}{r} 21\,{}^7/_{16} \\ -\;\;7\,{}^{12}/_{16} \\ \hline \end{array}$

4. $\begin{array}{r} {}^{27}/_{32} \\ -\,{}^{18}/_{32} \\ \hline \end{array}$

5. $\begin{array}{r} {}^7/_8 \\ -\,{}^2/_3 \\ \hline \end{array}$

6. $\begin{array}{r} 3\,{}^5/_8 \\ -\,1\,{}^3/_8 \\ \hline \end{array}$

7. $\begin{array}{r} 5\,{}^3/_7 \\ -\,1\,{}^6/_7 \\ \hline \end{array}$

8. $\begin{array}{r} 7 \\ -\,1\,{}^3/_4 \\ \hline \end{array}$

UNIT E

Math objective

Multiply fractions and mixed numbers.

Multiplication of fractions and mixed numbers

RULE:
1 Change mixed number to improper fraction.
2 Cancel if possible by dividing any top and bottom number by the largest number contained in each.
3 Multiply remaining top number to find top-number result.
4 Multiply bottom number to find bottom-number result.
5 Reduce answer to lowest terms.

EXAMPLE:

1 $1\,^4/_5 \times\, ^{15}/_{16} = \dfrac{\overset{1}{\cancel{4}}}{\underset{1}{\cancel{5}}} \times \dfrac{\overset{3}{\cancel{15}}}{\underset{4}{\cancel{16}}} = \,^3/_4$

2 $4^1/_2 \times 2^1/_4 = \dfrac{9}{2} \times \dfrac{9}{4} = \dfrac{81}{8} = 10^1/_8$

3 $6 \times\, ^3/_8 = \dfrac{6}{1} \times \dfrac{3}{8} = \dfrac{\overset{3}{\cancel{6}}}{1} \times \dfrac{3}{\underset{4}{\cancel{8}}} = \dfrac{9}{4} = 2^1/_4$

1E Worksheet

Multiply the following fractions and mixed numbers (reduce answer to lowest terms):

1. $^1/_3 \times\, ^2/_4 =$ 5. $^1/_5 \times\, ^1/_3 =$

2. $5^1/_2 \times 3^1/_8 =$ 6. $^3/_4 \times\, ^5/_8 =$

3. $1^3/_4 \times 3^1/_7 =$ 7. $^5/_6 \times 1^9/_{16} =$

4. $4 \times\, ^1/_8 =$ 8. $^5/_{100} \times 900 =$

UNIT F

Math objective

Divide fractions and mixed numbers.

Division of fractions and mixed numbers

RULE:
1. Change mixed number to improper fractions.
2. Turn the number after the ÷ (division) sign upside down.
3. Follow steps for multiplying and reduce any fractions.

EXAMPLE:

$$1 \quad \frac{1}{2} \div \frac{5}{8} = \frac{1}{2} \times \frac{8}{5} = \frac{8}{10} = \frac{4}{5}$$

$$2 \quad 8^3/_4 \div 15 = \frac{35}{4} \times \frac{1}{15} = \frac{\overset{7}{\cancel{35}}}{4} \times \frac{1}{\underset{3}{\cancel{15}}} = \frac{7}{12}$$

1F Worksheet

Divide the following fractions and mixed numbers:

1. $^2/_5 \div {}^5/_8 =$

2. $8^3/_4 \div 15 =$

3. $^3/_4 \div {}^1/_8 =$

4. $^1/_{16} \div {}^1/_4 =$

5. $^3/_4 \div 6 =$

6. $2 \div {}^1/_5 =$

7. $3^3/_8 \div 4^1/_2 =$

8. $^3/_5 \div {}^3/_8 =$

9

UNIT G

Math objective

Given two fractions, determine which is greater and which is smaller.

Value of fractions

RULE: The smaller the bottom number of a fraction, the greater it is in value. Make a whole number out of a fraction to see which one is larger.

EXAMPLE: $1/6$ is greater than $1/9$ because the bottom number is smaller.

RULE: To make a whole number out of the fraction $6/6$ means there are 6 parts to the whole number.

EXAMPLE:

$$\boxed{\frac{1}{6}\;\frac{1}{6}\;\frac{1}{6}\;\frac{1}{6}\;\frac{1}{6}\;\frac{1}{6}} = 6 \text{ parts} \qquad \text{Each } 1/6 \text{ part is larger than the } 1/9 \text{ part.}$$

$$\boxed{\frac{1}{9}\;\frac{1}{9}\;\frac{1}{9}\;\frac{1}{9}\;\frac{1}{9}\;\frac{1}{9}\;\frac{1}{9}\;\frac{1}{9}\;\frac{1}{9}} = 9 \text{ parts} \qquad \text{Each } 1/9 \text{ part is smaller than the } 1/6 \text{ part.}$$

Which would you rather have: $\dfrac{1}{6}$ or $\dfrac{1}{9}$ of your favorite pie?

1G Worksheet

Solve the following problems:

1. Which is greater: $1/3$ or $1/5$?

2. Which is smaller: $1/100$ or $1/150$?

3. Which is greater: $1/250$ or $1/300$?

4. Which is smaller: $1/6$ or $1/8$?

In the following three problems, *estimate* answers before beginning. This is a good habit to develop.

5. Doctor ordered gr $1/150$. On hand you have gr $1/200$ tablets. Will you need to give more or less than what is on hand?

6. On hand you have gr $1/150$ tablets. Doctor ordered gr $1/300$. Will you need to give more or less than what is on hand?

7. Doctor ordered gr $1/6$. You have on hand gr $1/4$ tablets. Will you need more or less than what is on hand?

UNIT H

Math objectives

1. *Distinguish among decimal fractions in tenths, hundredths, ten-thousandths, and hundred-thousandths.*
2. *Read whole numbers and decimal fractions.*

Value of decimals

A decimal fraction is a fraction whose denominator (bottom number) is 10, 100, 1000, 10,000, etc. It differs from a common fraction in that the denominator (bottom number) is *not* written but is expressed by the proper placement of the decimal point.

Observe the scale below. All whole numbers are to the left of the decimal point; all decimal fractions are to the right.

RULE: **1** All whole numbers are to the left of the decimal; all decimal fractions are to the right of the decimal point.

2 To read a decimal fraction, read the number to the right of the decimal and use the name that applies to "place value" of the *last* figure. All decimal fractions read with a *ths* on the end, except *half* and *thirds*.

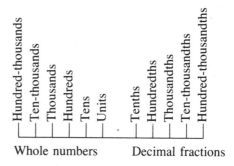

EXAMPLE: 0.257 = Two-hundred-fifty-seven thousand*ths*
0.2057 = Two-thousand-fifty-seven ten-thousand*ths*
0.20057 = Twenty-thousand-fifty-seven hundred-thousand*ths*

RULE: **3** To read a whole number and a fraction, the decimal point reads as an *and*.

EXAMPLE: 327.006 = Three hundred twenty-seven *and* six thousand*ths*

1H Worksheet

Read the following out loud:

1. 0.08   3. 0.0017   5. 0.0006

2. 0.092   4. 3287.467   6. 100.01

Express the following as decimal fractions:

7. Thirty-six hundredths   _____

8. Three thousandths   _____

9. Eight ten-thousandths   _____

10. Two and seventeen thousandths _____

11. Five hundredths   _____

12. Four and one tenth   _____

13. Twenty-four and two tenths   _____

UNIT I

Math objective

Divide decimals to third decimal place.

Division of decimals

RULE: 1 If divisor (number you are dividing by) is a whole number, divide as in the division of whole numbers. In the answer put the decimal in the same place as it is in the number to be divided.

2 If the divisor (number you are dividing by) is a decimal, make it a whole number by moving it to the end of the divisor. Move the decimal in the number being divided the same number of places.

EXAMPLE:

$$15 \div 6.2 = 6.2\overline{)15.0\,000}$$

$$
\begin{array}{r}
2.419 \\
6.2\,)\overline{15.0\,000} \\
12\ 4 \\
\hline
2\ 6\ 0 \\
2\ 4\ 8 \\
\hline
1\ 20 \\
62 \\
\hline
580 \\
558 \\
\hline
22
\end{array}
$$

1I Worksheet _____

Divide the following and carry to the *third* decimal place if necessary:

1. $158.4 \div 48$

2. $200 \div 6.0$

3. $15.06 \div 6$

4. $79.4 \div 0.87$

5. $670.8 \div 0.78$

6. $78.6 \div 2.43$

7. $26.78 \div 8.2$

8. $266.5 \div 5.78$

9. $10.80 \div 6.5$

10. $76.53 \div 10$

UNIT J

Math objective

Add decimals.

Addition of decimals

RULE: **1** Write decimals in column; keep decimal points one under the other.
2 Add as in whole numbers.
3 Put the decimal point in the same place as in the number to be added.

EXAMPLE:

$$
\begin{array}{r} 0.8 \\ +0.5 \\ \hline 1.3 \end{array}
\qquad
\begin{array}{r} 3.27 \\ +0.06 \\ \hline 3.33 \end{array}
$$

1J Worksheet

Add the following decimals:

1. $0.8 + 0.5 =$

2. $3.27 + 0.06 + 2 =$

3. $5.01 + 2.999 =$

4. $15.6 + 0.19 + 200 =$

5. $210.79 + 2 + 68.4 =$

6. $88.6 + 576.46 + 79.0 =$

7. $6.77 + 102 + 88.3 =$

8. $79.4 + 68.44 + 3.00 =$

9. $10.56 + 356.4 =$

10. $99.7 + 293.23 =$

UNIT K

Math objective

Multiply decimals.

Multiplication of decimals

RULE: 1 Multiply as in multiplying whole numbers.
2 Find the total number of decimal places in the multiplier *and* in the number to be multiplied.
3 Start from the right and count off the same number of places in the answer.
4 If the answer does not have enough places, supply as many zeros as needed.

EXAMPLE: $2.6 \times 0.0002 = $ $\quad$ 2.6 (1 decimal place)
$\underline{\times 0.0002 \text{ (4 decimal places)}}$
0.00052 (5 decimal places starting at the right in the answer)

1K Worksheet

Multiply the following decimals:

1. $3.14 \times 0.002 = $

2. $95.26 \times 1.125 = $

3. $100 \times 0.5 = $

4. $2.14 \times 0.03 = $

5. $36.8 \times 70.1 = $

6. $203.7 \times 28 = $

7. $88 \times 90.1 = $

8. $2.76 \times 0.003 = $

9. $54.5 \times 21 = $

10. $200 \times 0.2 = $

UNIT L

Math objective

Subtract decimals.

Subtraction of decimals

RULE: **1** Write decimals in a column, keeping the decimal points under each other.
2 Subtract as in whole numbers.
3 Place the decimal point in the answer directly under the decimal point in the sums to be added (zeros can be added *after* the decimal point without changing the value).

EXAMPLE: $0.6 - 0.524 =$ $\begin{array}{r} 0.600 \\ -0.524 \\ \hline 0.076 \end{array}$

1L Worksheet

Subtract the following decimals:

1. $98.4 - 66.50 =$

2. $108.56 - 5.40 =$

3. $0.450 - 0.367 =$

4. $21.78 - 19.88 =$

5. $266.44 - 0.56 =$

6. $7.066 - 0.200 =$

7. $34.678 - 0.502 =$

8. $78.567 - 6.77 =$

9. $1.723 - 0.683 =$

10. $0.8100 - 0.6701 =$

UNIT M

Math objectives

1. *Change decimals to fractions.*
2. *Reduce fractions to lowest terms.*

Changing decimals to fractions

RULE: **1** The numbers to the *right* of the decimal can be written as a fraction because they are only part of the whole number.

2 REMEMBER: The first number past the decimal to the *right* is ten*ths* (10), the second is hundred*ths* (100), the third is thousand*ths* (1000), the fourth is ten-thousand*ths* (10,000), and so on.

3 So if your problem has 3 numbers to the *right* of the decimal, just remove the decimal and put the number over 1000.

EXAMPLE: **1** 0.375 has 3 numbers to the *right* of the decimal. To make a fraction out of 0.375 and also get rid of the decimal, just put it over 1000.

0.375 written as a fraction is $^{375}/_{1000}$.

It's easy to remember: 3 numbers on top and 3 zeros on the bottom.

2 0.90 written as a fraction is $^{90}/_{100}$.

The idea is the same as above: 2 numbers on top and 2 zeros on the bottom.

1M Worksheet

Work problems and reduce to lowest terms:

1. 0.40 =

2. 0.8 =

3. 0.250 =

4. 4.08 =

5. 1.32 =

6. 0.500 =

7. 0.750 =

8. 0.20 =

9. 0.65 =

10. 0.700 =

UNIT N

Math objective

Change fractions to decimals.

Changing common fractions to decimals

RULE: 1 Divide the top number by the bottom number and place the decimal point in the proper position.

EXAMPLE: $2/5 = $

$$\begin{array}{r} 0.40 = 0.4 \\ 5\overline{)2.00} \\ \underline{2.0} \\ 0 \end{array}$$

1N Worksheet

Carry out division to *third* decimal place:

1. $19/100 =$

2. $9/7 =$

3. $59/16 =$

4. $1/5 =$

5. $2/3 =$

6. $1/2 =$

7. $1/12 =$

8. $6/8 =$

9. $15/200 =$

10. $20/8 =$

UNIT O

Math objectives

1. *Change percent to fraction.*
2. *Convert fraction to decimal.*
3. *Change percent to decimal.*
4. *Convert decimal to percent.*

Percentages, decimals, and fractions

Percent

The term *percent* and its symbol (%) mean hundred*ths*. A percent number is a fraction whose top number is already known and whose bottom is *always* understood to be 100.

Changing a percent to a fraction

EXAMPLE: **1** 5% written as a fraction is $^5/_{100}$.

REMEMBER: The top number is the percent and the bottom number is always 100. Drop the percent sign when converting 5% to $^5/_{100}$.

2 $^1/_2$% is written as a fraction $\dfrac{^1/_2}{.100}$. You cannot leave the problem like this. $\dfrac{^1/_2}{100}$ means $^1/_2 \div 100 = ^1/_2 \times ^1/_{100} = ^1/_{200}$. The problem is completed when $\dfrac{^1/_2}{100} = ^1/_2 \times ^1/_{100} = ^1/_{200}$.

Converting a fraction to a decimal

RULE: **1** The fraction $^5/_{100}$ can be made into a decimal by dividing the bottom number into the top number.

EXAMPLE: **1** To change $^5/_{100}$ into a decimal means $5 \div 100$.

$$100)\overline{5.00} \quad \begin{array}{c} .05 \end{array}$$

Don't forget the decimal point.

$$\underline{5\ 00}$$

2 Change $^1/_{200}$ to a decimal. Divide the bottom number into the top number.

$$1 \div 200 = 200)\overline{1.000} \quad \begin{array}{c} .005 \end{array}$$

$$\underline{1\ 000}$$

Changing a percent to a decimal

RULE: **1** A percent number can be changed to a decimal by having its decimal point moved 2 places to the *left* to signify hundred*ths*.

EXAMPLE: **1** 5% written as a decimal is 0.05.
REMEMBER: Move the decimal 2 places to the *left* and drop the % sign.

2 0.5% written as a decimal is 0.005.
REMEMBER: Move the decimal 2 places to the *left* and drop the % sign.

Converting a decimal to a percent

RULE: **1** The only thing you must do is to move the decimal point 2 places to the *right* and add the percent sign.

EXAMPLE: **1** 0.05 is a decimal. To make it a percent, move the decimal point 2 places to the *right* and add the % sign. Therefore 0.05 = 5%.
2 0.005 = 0.5% or $\frac{1}{2}$%

1O Worksheet

	Fraction	Decimal	Percent
1.			$66\frac{2}{3}$%
2.	$\frac{1}{2}$		
3.			6.5%
4.	$\frac{1}{12}$		
5.	$\frac{3}{1000}$		
6.		0.10	
7.			250%
8.		0.35	
9.	$\frac{4}{5}$		
10.			78%

If you are having difficulty with fractions, decimals, or percents, review Section 1, Unit O, or see your instructor.

UNIT P

Math objective

Find percent.

Finding the percentage

RULE: **1** Change the percent to a decimal or common fraction.
            2 *Multiply* the number by this decimal.

EXAMPLE: 23% of 64 = 64 × 0.23 = 14.72

1P Worksheet

1. 114% of 240 =   5. 28% of 50 =   9. 10% of 520 =

2. 2% of 1500 =   6. 9% of 200 =   10. 3% of 40.80 =

3. ½% of 9328 =   7. 120% of 400 =

4. ⅓% of 930 =   8. 5% of 105.80 =

Section 1 GENERAL MATHEMATICS ANSWER SHEETS

1A Answer sheet

1. 1
2. $3^{1}/_{4}$
3. 3
4. $1^{5}/_{9}$

5. $5^{2}/_{3}$
6. 4
7. $1^{3}/_{4}$

8. $1^{7}/_{8}$
9. 3
10. $6^{5}/_{6}$

1B Answer sheet

1. $^{6}/_{5}$
2. $^{5}/_{4}$
3. $^{49}/_{3}$
4. $^{43}/_{12}$

5. $^{68}/_{5}$
6. $^{35}/_{8}$
7. $^{23}/_{6}$

8. $^{21}/_{8}$
9. $^{63}/_{6}$
10. $^{377}/_{3}$

1C Answer sheet

1.
$$\begin{array}{r} ^{1}/_{5} \\ +^{2}/_{5} \\ \hline ^{3}/_{5} \end{array}$$

2.
$$\begin{array}{r} ^{3}/_{5} = \ ^{9}/_{15} \\ +^{2}/_{3} = \ ^{10}/_{15} \\ \hline ^{19}/_{15} = 1^{4}/_{15} \end{array}$$

3.
$$\begin{array}{r} 6^{1}/_{6} = \ 6\ ^{4}/_{24} \\ +9^{5}/_{8} = \ 9^{15}/_{24} \\ \hline 15^{19}/_{24} \end{array}$$

4.
$$\begin{array}{r} 1^{3}/_{8} = \ 1^{15}/_{40} \\ +9^{9}/_{10} = \ 9^{36}/_{40} \\ \hline 10^{51}/_{40} = 11^{11}/_{40} \end{array}$$

5.
$$\begin{array}{r} ^{1}/_{8} = \ ^{9}/_{72} \\ ^{1}/_{4} = \ ^{18}/_{72} \\ +^{2}/_{9} = \ ^{16}/_{72} \\ \hline ^{43}/_{72} \end{array}$$

6.
$$\begin{array}{r} ^{7}/_{9} = \ ^{70}/_{90} \\ ^{4}/_{5} = \ ^{72}/_{90} \\ +^{9}/_{10} = \ ^{81}/_{90} \\ \hline ^{223}/_{90} = 2^{43}/_{90} \end{array}$$

7.
$$\begin{array}{r} 3^{1}/_{4} \\ +9^{3}/_{4} \\ \hline 12^{4}/_{4} = 13 \end{array}$$

8.
$$\begin{array}{r} 8^{2}/_{5} = \ 8\ ^{4}/_{10} \\ 14^{7}/_{10} = 14\ ^{7}/_{10} \\ + \ 9^{9}/_{10} = \ 9\ ^{9}/_{10} \\ \hline 31^{20}/_{10} = 33 \end{array}$$

1D Answer sheet

1. $\frac{4}{5} = \frac{8}{10}$
   $-\frac{1}{2} = \frac{5}{10}$
   $\frac{3}{10}$

2. $7\frac{16}{24} = 7\frac{16}{24}$
   $-3\frac{1}{8} = 3\frac{3}{24}$
   $4\frac{13}{24}$

3. $21\frac{7}{16} = 20\frac{23}{16}$ Must borrow from whole number.
   $-7\frac{12}{16} = 7\frac{12}{16}$
   $13\frac{11}{16}$

4. $\frac{27}{32}$
   $-\frac{18}{32}$
   $\frac{9}{32}$

5. $\frac{7}{8} = \frac{21}{24}$
   $-\frac{2}{3} = \frac{16}{24}$
   $\frac{5}{24}$

6. $3\frac{5}{8}$
   $-1\frac{3}{8}$
   $2\frac{2}{8} = 2\frac{1}{4}$

7. $5\frac{3}{7} = 4\frac{10}{7}$ Must borrow from whole number.
   $-1\frac{6}{7} = 1\frac{6}{7}$
   $3\frac{4}{7}$

8. $7 = 6\frac{4}{4}$ Must borrow from whole number.
   $-1\frac{3}{4} = 1\frac{3}{4}$
   $5\frac{1}{4}$

1E Answer sheet

1. $^1/_3 \times {}^2/_4 = {}^2/_{12} = {}^1/_6$

2. $5^1/_2 \times 3^1/_8 = {}^{11}/_2 \times {}^{25}/_8 = {}^{275}/_{16} = 275 \div 16 = 17^3/_{16}$

3. $1^3/_4 \times 3^1/_7 = \dfrac{\overset{1}{\cancel{7}}}{4} \times \dfrac{22}{\underset{1}{\cancel{7}}} = {}^{22}/_4 = 22 \div 4 = 5^1/_2$

4. $4 \times {}^1/_8 = \dfrac{\overset{1}{\cancel{4}}}{\underset{2}{\cancel{8}}} = {}^1/_2$

5. $^1/_5 \times {}^1/_3 = {}^1/_{15}$

6. $^3/_4 \times {}^5/_8 = {}^{15}/_{32}$

7. $^5/_6 \times 1^9/_{16} = {}^5/_6 \times {}^{25}/_{16} = {}^{125}/_{96} = 125 \div 96 = 1^{29}/_{96}$

8. $^5/_{100} \times 900 = \dfrac{5}{\underset{1}{\cancel{100}}} \times \dfrac{\overset{9}{\cancel{900}}}{1} = 45$

1F Answer sheet

1. $^2/_5 \div {}^5/_8 = {}^2/_5 \times {}^8/_5 = {}^{16}/_{25}$

2. $8^3/_4 \div 15 = \dfrac{\overset{7}{\cancel{35}}}{4} \times \dfrac{1}{\underset{3}{\cancel{15}}} = \dfrac{7}{12}$

3. $^3/_4 \div {}^1/_8 = \dfrac{3}{\underset{1}{\cancel{4}}} \times \dfrac{\overset{2}{\cancel{8}}}{1} = 6$

4. $^1/_{16} \div {}^1/_4 = \dfrac{1}{\underset{4}{\cancel{16}}} \times \dfrac{\overset{1}{\cancel{4}}}{1} = {}^1/_4$

5. $^3/_4 \div 6 = \dfrac{\overset{1}{\cancel{3}}}{4} \times \dfrac{1}{\underset{2}{\cancel{6}}} = {}^1/_8$

6. $2 \div {}^1/_5 = {}^2/_1 \times {}^5/_1 = 10$

7. $3^3/_8 \div 4^1/_2 = {}^{27}/_8 \div {}^9/_2 = \dfrac{\overset{3}{\cancel{27}}}{\underset{4}{\cancel{8}}} \times \dfrac{\overset{1}{\cancel{2}}}{\underset{1}{\cancel{9}}} = {}^3/_4$

8. $^3/_5 \div {}^3/_8 = \dfrac{\overset{1}{\cancel{3}}}{5} \times \dfrac{8}{\underset{1}{\cancel{3}}} = {}^8/_5 = 1^3/_5$

1G Answer sheet

1. $1/3$
2. $1/150$
3. $1/250$
4. $1/8$
5. More
6. Less
7. Less

1H Answer sheet

1. Eight hundredths
2. Ninety-two thousandths
3. Seventeen ten-thousandths
4. Three thousand two hundred eighty-seven and four hundred sixty-seven thousandths
5. Six ten-thousandths
6. One hundred and one hundredth
7. 0.36
8. 0.003
9. 0.0008
10. 2.017
11. 0.05
12. 4.1
13. 24.2

```
            3.3                      8 60.                      1.661
1.  48)158.4            5.  0.78)670.80.          9.  6.5)10.8.000
        144                      624                          6 5
         14 4                     46 8                        4 30
         14 4                     46 8                        3 90
                                                              4 00
                                                              3 90
           3 3.333                32.345                       100
2.  6.0)200.0.000       6.  2.43)78.60.000                      65
        180                      72 9
         20 0                     5 70
         18 0                     4 86
          2 00                    84 0                         7.653
          1 80                    72 9         10.  10)76.530
           2 00                   11 10                         70
           1 80                    9 72                         6 5
            200                   1 380                         6 0
            180                   1 215                          53
                                                                50
                                                                30
         2.51                    3.265                          30
3.  6)15.06             7.  8.2)26.7.800
        12                       24 6
         3 0                      2 1 8
         3 0                      1 6 4
          6                       5 40
          6                       4 92
                                  480
                                  410
           91.264
4.  0.87)79.40.000                46.107
         78 3          8.  5.78)266.50.000
          1 10                   231 2
           87                    35 30
           23 0                  34 68
           17 4                   62 0
            5 60                   57 8
            5 22                  4 200
             380                  4 046
             348
```

1J Answer sheet

1.
```
  0.8
+0.5
  1.3
```

2.
```
  3.27
  0.06
+2.
  5.33
```

3.
```
  5.01
+2.999
  8.009
```

4.
```
   15.6
    0.19
+200.
  215.79
```

5.
```
  210.79
    2.
+  68.4
  281.19
```

6.
```
   88.6
  576.46
+  79.
  744.06
```

7.
```
    6.77
  102.
+  88.3
  197.07
```

8.
```
   79.4
   68.44
+  3.
  150.84
```

9.
```
   10.56
+356.4
  366.96
```

10.
```
   99.7
+293.23
  392.93
```

1K Answer sheet

1. $\begin{array}{r} 3.14 \\ \times 0.002 \\ \hline 0.00628 \end{array}$ You do not have to multiply zeros. Count 5 places in from the right, adding zeros where needed.

2. $\begin{array}{r} 95.26 \\ \times 1.125 \\ \hline 47630 \\ 19052 \\ 9526 \\ 9526 \\ \hline 107.16750 \end{array}$ Count 5 decimal places in from the right.

3. $\begin{array}{r} 0.5 \\ \times 100 \\ \hline 50.0 \end{array}$ Count 1 decimal place in from the right.

4. $\begin{array}{r} 2.14 \\ \times 0.03 \\ \hline 0.0642 \end{array}$ Count 4 decimal places in from the right, adding zeros as needed.

5. $\begin{array}{r} 36.8 \\ \times 70.1 \\ \hline 368 \\ 2576 \\ \hline 2579.68 \end{array}$

6. $\begin{array}{r} 203.7 \\ \times 28 \\ \hline 16296 \\ 4074 \\ \hline 5703.6 \end{array}$

7. $\begin{array}{r} 90.1 \\ \times 88 \\ \hline 7208 \\ 7208 \\ \hline 7928.8 \end{array}$

8. $\begin{array}{r} 2.76 \\ \times 0.003 \\ \hline 0.00828 \end{array}$

9. $\begin{array}{r} 54.5 \\ \times 21 \\ \hline 545 \\ 1090 \\ \hline 1144.5 \end{array}$

10. $\begin{array}{r} 200 \\ \times 0.2 \\ \hline 40.0 \end{array}$

1L Answer sheet

1.
$$\begin{array}{r} 98.4 \\ -66.50 \\ \hline 31.90 \end{array}$$

2.
$$\begin{array}{r} 108.56 \\ -\;\;\;5.40 \\ \hline 103.16 \end{array}$$

3.
$$\begin{array}{r} 0.450 \\ -0.367 \\ \hline 0.083 \end{array}$$

4.
$$\begin{array}{r} 21.78 \\ -19.88 \\ \hline 1.90 \end{array}$$

5.
$$\begin{array}{r} 266.44 \\ -\;\;\;0.56 \\ \hline 265.88 \end{array}$$

6.
$$\begin{array}{r} 7.066 \\ -0.200 \\ \hline 6.866 \end{array}$$

7.
$$\begin{array}{r} 34.678 \\ -\;\;0.502 \\ \hline 34.176 \end{array}$$

8.
$$\begin{array}{r} 78.567 \\ -\;\;6.77 \\ \hline 71.797 \end{array}$$

9.
$$\begin{array}{r} 1.723 \\ -0.683 \\ \hline 1.040 \end{array}$$

10.
$$\begin{array}{r} 0.8100 \\ -0.6701 \\ \hline 0.1399 \end{array}$$

1M Answer sheet

1. $\dfrac{4\cancel{0}}{10\cancel{0}} = \dfrac{2}{5}$

2. $\dfrac{8}{10} = \dfrac{4}{5}$

3. $\dfrac{25\cancel{0}}{100\cancel{0}} = \dfrac{1}{4}$

4. $4\dfrac{08}{100} = 4^2/_{25}$

5. $1\dfrac{32}{100} = \dfrac{8}{25} = 1^8/_{25}$

6. $\dfrac{5\cancel{0}\cancel{0}}{100\cancel{0}\cancel{0}} = \dfrac{1}{2}$

7. $\dfrac{75\cancel{0}}{100\cancel{0}} = \dfrac{3}{4}$

8. $\dfrac{2\cancel{0}}{10\cancel{0}} = \dfrac{1}{5}$

9. $\dfrac{65}{100} = \dfrac{13}{20}$

10. $\dfrac{7\cancel{0}\cancel{0}}{100\cancel{0}\cancel{0}} = \dfrac{7}{10}$

1.
$$100\overline{)19.00}$$ → 0.19
$$\underline{10\ 0}$$
$$9\ 00$$
$$\underline{9\ 00}$$

2.
$$7\overline{)9.00}$$ → 1.285
$$\underline{7}$$
$$2\ 0$$
$$\underline{1\ 4}$$
$$60$$
$$\underline{56}$$
$$40$$
$$\underline{35}$$

3. $5^9/_{16} = 5 \times 16 + 9 = {}^{89}/_{16}$

$$16\overline{)89.000}$$ → 5.562¹/₂
$$\underline{80}$$
$$9\ 0$$
$$\underline{8\ 0}$$
$$1\ 00$$
$$\underline{96}$$
$$40$$
$$\underline{32}$$
$$8$$

4.
$$5\overline{)1.0}$$ → 0.2
$$\underline{1.0}$$

5.
$$3\overline{)2.000}$$ → 0.666
$$\underline{1\ 8}$$
$$20$$
$$\underline{18}$$
$$20$$
$$\underline{18}$$

6.
$$2\overline{)1.0}$$ → 0.5
$$\underline{1.0}$$

7.
$$12\overline{)1.000}$$ → 0.083
$$\underline{96}$$
$$40$$
$$\underline{36}$$

8.
$$8\overline{)6.00}$$ → 0.75
$$\underline{5\ 6}$$
$$40$$
$$\underline{40}$$

9.
$$200\overline{)15.000}$$ → 0.075
$$\underline{14\ 00}$$
$$1\ 000$$
$$\underline{1\ 000}$$

10.
$$8\overline{)20.0}$$ → 2.5
$$\underline{16}$$
$$4\ 0$$
$$\underline{4\ 0}$$

1O Answer sheet

1. Fraction: $^2/_3$
   Decimal: 0.67

2. Decimal: 0.5
   Percent: 50%

3. Fraction: $^{13}/_{200}$
   Decimal: 0.065

4. Decimal: 0.0833
   Percent: 8.33%

5. Decimal: 0.003
   Percent: 0.3%

6. Fraction: $^1/_{10}$
   Percent: 10%

7. Fraction: $^{250}/_{100} = {}^5/_2$
   Decimal: 2.5

8. Fraction: $^7/_{20}$
   Percent: 35%

9. Decimal: 0.8
   Percent: 80%

10. Fraction: $^{78}/_{100} = {}^{39}/_{50}$
    Decimal: 0.78

1. $\begin{array}{r} 240 \\ \times 1.14 \\ \hline 960 \\ 240 \\ 240 \\ \hline 273.60 \end{array}$

2. $\begin{array}{r} 1500 \\ \times .02 \\ \hline 30.00 \end{array}$

3. $\dfrac{^{1}/_{2}}{100} = \dfrac{1}{2} \div \dfrac{100}{1} = \dfrac{1}{2} \times \dfrac{1}{100} = \dfrac{1}{200} = 200\overline{)1.000}^{\,.005}$
    $\begin{array}{r} 9328 \\ \times .005 \\ \hline 46.640 \end{array}$ *Answer*

4. $\dfrac{^{1}/_{3}}{100} = \dfrac{1}{3} \div \dfrac{100}{1} = \dfrac{1}{3} \times \dfrac{1}{100} = \dfrac{1}{300} = 300\overline{)1.000}^{\,.003}$
    $\begin{array}{r} 900 \\ \hline 100 \end{array}$
    $\begin{array}{r} 930 \\ \times .003 \\ \hline 2.790 \end{array}$ *Answer*

5. $\begin{array}{r} 50 \\ \times .28 \\ \hline 400 \\ 100 \\ \hline 14.00 \end{array}$

6. $\begin{array}{r} 200 \\ \times .09 \\ \hline 18.00 \end{array}$

7. $\begin{array}{r} 400 \\ \times 1.20 \\ \hline 8000 \\ 400 \\ \hline 480.00 \end{array}$

8. $\begin{array}{r} 105.80 \\ \times .05 \\ \hline 5.2900 \end{array}$

9. $\begin{array}{r} 520 \\ \times .10 \\ \hline 52.00 \end{array}$

10. $\begin{array}{r} 40.80 \\ \times .03 \\ \hline 1.2240 \end{array}$

Section 1 GENERAL MATH QUIZ

Change to whole or mixed numbers:

1. $^{34}/_6$

2. $^{48}/_7$

Change to improper fractions:

3. $13^3/_5$

4. $3^5/_6$

Find the lowest common bottom number in the following fractions:

5. $^{17}/_{20}$ and $^4/_5$

6. $^7/_8$ and $^3/_5$

Add the following numbers:

7. $^1/_{18}$, $^1/_4$, and $^2/_9$

8. $5^1/_8$, $1^1/_4$, and $4^1/_2$

Subtract the following:

9. $^7/_8 - ^2/_3$

10. $6^2/_4 - 5^1/_2$

Multiply the following:

11. $^1/_5 \times ^1/_3$

12. $^5/_6 \times ^2/_8$

Divide the following:

13. $^3/_4 \div ^1/_8$

14. $3^3/_8 \div 4^1/_2$

Express the following ratios as fractions reduced to lowest terms (numbers):

15. 2:500

16. 2:13

Write the following as decimals:

17. Thirty-six hundredths _____

18. Two and seventeen thousandths _____

Add the following:

19. 5.01 + 2.999

20. 36.87 + 8.26 + 15.84

Subtract the following:

21. 4 − 0.176

22. 0.41 − 0.2538

Multiply the following:

23. 0.0005 × 0.02

24. 5 × 0.7

Divide the following and carry to the third decimal place:

25. 158.4 ÷ 48

26. 79.4 ÷ 0.87

Change the following to decimals:

27. $^{57}/_{48}$

28. $8^1/_{16}$

Solve the following percents:

29. 24% of 52

30. $6^1/_4$% of 9328

Change the following decimals to fractions:

31. 0.400

32. 0.285

33. Write 43% as a decimal and as a fraction.

34. Write $^1/_{10}$ as a decimal and as a percent.

Section 1 General math quiz answer sheet _____

1. $5^2/_3$
2. $6^6/_7$
3. $^{68}/_5$
4. $^{23}/_6$
5. 20
6. 40
7. $^{19}/_{36}$
8. $10^7/_8$
9. $^5/_{24}$
10. 1
11. $^1/_{15}$
12. $^5/_{24}$

13. 6
14. $^3/_4$
15. $^1/_{250}$
16. $^2/_{13}$
17. 0.36
18. 2.017
19. 8.009
20. 60.97
21. 3.824
22. 0.1562
23. 0.000010

24. 3.5
25. 3.300
26. 91.264
27. 1.1875
28. 8.0625
29. 12.48
30. 583.00
31. $^2/_5$
32. $^{57}/_{200}$
33. 0.43 and $^{43}/_{100}$
34. 0.10 and 10%

SECTION 2

Ratio and proportion

UNIT A

Math objectives

1. *Express ratios as fractions.*
2. *Reduce fractions to lowest numerical terms.*

Ratio

RULE: A ratio indicates the relationship of one quantity to another. It indicates *division* and may be expressed in fraction form.

EXAMPLE: $\frac{1}{3}$ may be expressed as a ratio $1:3$.

2A Worksheet

Express the following ratios as fractions reduced to lowest terms:

1. $2:4$

2. $4:6$

3. $2:500$

4. $6:1000$

5. $43:86$

6. $2:13$

7. $7:49$

8. $1:5$

9. $1:150$

10. $4:100$

Section 2 answer sheets begin on p. 46.

UNIT B

Math objective

Solve ratio/proportion problems for x.

Proportion

A proportion shows the relationship between two equal ratios. A proportion may be expressed as $3:5::6:10$ or $3:5 = 6:10$.

To solve the ratio and proportion problems, just do this:

RULE:
1 Multiply the two inside numbers.
2 Multiply the two outside numbers.
3 The answers should be the same.

EXAMPLE:
$3:5::6:10$

multiply

Multiply the two *inside* numbers: $5 \times 6 = 30$
Multiply the two *outside* numbers: $3 \times 10 = 30$

How to solve the problem when one of the numbers is unknown or x

Always multiply the x first and put it on the *left* side of the equation.

EXAMPLE:
$3:5::x:10$

Multiply inside numbers: $5x$. Multiply outside numbers: $3 \times 10 = 30$. The equation will now look like this: $5x = 30$.

4 Now you must get x to stand alone. Cancel it out, and you will never go wrong. Whatever you do to one side you must do to the other to keep them equal. Canceling out eliminates the chance of dividing the wrong sides into each other. The end product of canceling out is a fraction, that is: $^{30}/_5$.

A fraction means that the bottom number is always divided into the top number.

EXAMPLE:
This cancels the 5 out: $\dfrac{\cancel{5}x}{\cancel{5}} = \dfrac{30}{5}$

5 The only part of the problem left unsolved is $^{30}/_5$. As you know, $^{30}/_5$ means $30 \div 5 = 6$; so $x = 6$.

Put the entire problem together, following the five steps outlined above. Remember to always put x on the *left*-hand side.

multiply
$3:5::x:10$ or
multiply

$5x = 30$

$5x = 30$

What you do to one side of the equation you must do to the other. This cancels out the 5 and leaves x.

$$\frac{\cancel{5}x}{\cancel{5}} = \frac{30}{5} \qquad \text{This means } 30 \div 5 \text{ or } 5\overline{)30}^{\,6}$$

$$x = 6 \qquad\qquad\qquad\qquad \frac{30}{0}$$

How do you know your answer is correct?

To *prove* your answer, just substitute the answer for the x in the problem, multiply the inside numbers together, and then multiply the outside numbers together.

EXAMPLE: PROOF: $3:5::6:10$

$$5 \times 6 = 30$$
$$3 \times 10 = 30$$

Now you are ready to solve for x.

2B Worksheet

Solve the following problems for x:

1. $^{1}/_{2}:x::1:8$

2. $9:x::5:300$

3. $^{1}/_{1000}:^{1}/_{100}::x:60$

4. $^{1}/_{4}:500::x:1000$

5. $36:12::^{1}/_{100}:x$

6. $6:24::0.75:x$

7. $x:600::4:120$

8. $0.7:70::x:1000$

9. $9:27::300:x$

10. $6:12::^{1}/_{4}:x$

UNIT C

2C Worksheet

<small>REMEMBER</small>: Multiply two inside numbers, multiply two outside numbers, put x on the *left*.

Solve for x:

1. $^1/_{200} : x :: 1 : 800$

2. $15 : 30 :: x : 12$

3. $^1/_{1000} : ^1/_{100} :: x : 30$

4. $6 : 12 :: 0.25 : x$

5. $300 : 5 :: x : ^1/_{60}$

6. $^1/_{150} : ^1/_{200} :: 2 : x$

7. $^1/_2 : ^1/_6 :: ^1/_4 : x$

8. $7.5 : 12 :: x : 28$

9. $15 : x :: 1.5 : 10$

UNIT D

Math objective

Solve verbal and numerical ratio/proportion problems for x.

Ratio and proportion: how to set up

RULE:
1 To set up a ratio and proportion, you must always put on the *left*-hand side what you already *have* or what you already *know*.

2 On the *right*-hand side you will put your *x* or what you *want* to know.

3 Each side of the equation is set up the *same way*.

EXAMPLE: Apples : *Pears* :: Apples : *x Pears*

RULE:
4 Multiply the two inside numbers. Multiply the two outside numbers.

5 Always put *x* on the *left*.

6 Prove all answers and label.

EXAMPLE: PROBLEM: You wish to make a floral bouquet of 6 daffodils for every 4 roses. How many daffodils will you use for 30 roses?

Know   Want to know

6 daffodils : 4 roses :: *x* daffodils : 30 roses   PROOF: $4 \times 45 = 180$

$$\frac{4x}{4} = \frac{180}{4} = 180 \div 4 = 45$$ $6 \times 30 = 180$

Left
$4x = 180$

$x = 45$ daffodils

2D Worksheet

Problems to set up and prove:

1. You have a recipe for cocoa—4 scoops make 6 cups of cocoa. You want to make 18 cups for a party. How many scoops of cocoa? Set up a proportion:

2. You are making coffee, and 7 scoops make 8 cups. How many scoops make 40 cups?

3. You have to make a fruit basket with 6 bananas for every 9 apples. How many bananas for 72 apples?

4. Doctor ordered 450 mg of aspirin. On hand you have 300 mg in 1 tablet. How many tablets will you give?

5. You wish to plant 8 bushes for every 2 trees in your yard. How many bushes for 36 trees? (Estimate and prove.)

6. Doctor ordered 4 cups of All-Bran every day. How many days would it take to consume 84 cups of All-Bran? (Estimate and prove.)

7. It takes 4 cups of flour to make 3 loaves of bread. How many loaves of bread can be made from 24 cups of flour?

UNIT E

Math objectives

1. *Solve one-step ratio/proportion problems.*
2. *Estimate answers.*
3. *Prove answers.*

Ratio and proportion: how to set up

RULE:
1 You already know that what you *have* or what you know goes on the *left*-hand side of the equation. What you want to know goes on the *right*-hand side; so this will be the side for the *x,* or unknown.
2 Remember that both sides of the equation *must be* set up the same way.

EXAMPLE:
Make a necklace that has 19 blue beads for every 1 yellow bead. How many blue beads are needed if you have 8 yellow beads?
(Prove your answer.)

Have   **Want to know**

19 blue beads:1 yellow bead::*x* blue beads:8 yellow beads
— multiply —
— multiply —

1*x* = 152 blue beads needed   PROOF: $19 \times 8 = 152$
                                                                    $1 \times 152 = 152$

2E Worksheet

Work problems and prove:

1. Doctor ordered 40 mg of aspirin. You have on hand 5 mg tablets. How many tablets will you give? **a,** Will you give *more* or *less* than what you have on hand? **b,** How many tablets will you give? Prove your answer and label.

2. Ordered is ¼ gr of codeine. You have on hand ⅙ gr tablets. **a,** Will you give *more* or *less* than what you have on hand? **b,** Set up proportion and prove.

3. Doctor ordered $\frac{1}{6}$ gr of morphine. You have on hand $\frac{1}{8}$ gr in 1 tablet. **a,** Will you give *more* or *less* of what you have? **b,** Do your work and prove.

4. The doctor tells you to drink 3 glasses of H_2O and eat 2 apples every day. How many apples will you have eaten when you have drunk 24 glasses of water?

5. If you were going to give all the teachers 6 pens for every 8 pencils, how many pens would you give for 72 pencils?

6. If you were making an omelet with $\frac{1}{2}$ tsp. of salt for every 3 eggs, how much salt would you use for 30 eggs?

7. If your coffeemaker makes 8 cups of coffee for every 7 scoops of coffee, how many scoops would you need to make 24 cups of coffee?

Section 2 RATIO AND PROPORTION ANSWER SHEETS

2A Answer sheet

1. $^2/_4 = ^1/_2$
2. $^4/_6 = ^2/_3$
3. $^2/_{500} = ^1/_{250}$
4. $^6/_{1000} = ^3/_{500}$

5. $^{43}/_{86} = ^1/_2$
6. $^2/_{13}$
7. $^7/_{49} = ^1/_7$

8. $^1/_5$
9. $^1/_{150}$
10. $^4/_{100} = ^1/_{25}$

2B Answer sheet

REMEMBER: Always put x on the left.

1. $^1/_2 : x :: 1 : 8$

   $1x = ^1/_2 \times 8$

   $x = ^1/_2 \times ^8/_1 = 4$

   $x = 4$

   PROOF: $4 \times 1 = 4$

   $^1/_2 \times 8 = 4$

2. $9 : x :: 5 : 300$

   $5x = 9 \times 300$

   $5x = 2700$

   $\dfrac{5x}{5} = \dfrac{2700}{5} = 2700 \div 5 = 540$

   $x = 540$

   PROOF: $540 \times 5 = 2700$

   $9 \times 300 = 2700$

3. $^1/_{1000} : ^1/_{100} :: x : 60$

   $^1/_{100}x = ^1/_{1000} \times 60$

   $\dfrac{1}{100}x = \dfrac{1}{1000} \times \dfrac{60}{1} = \dfrac{1}{50} \times \dfrac{3}{1} = \dfrac{3}{50}$

   $\dfrac{^1/_{100}x}{^1/_{100}} = \dfrac{^3/_{50}}{^1/_{100}} = \dfrac{3}{50} \div \dfrac{1}{100} = \dfrac{3}{50} \times \dfrac{100}{1} = 6$

   $x = 6$

   PROOF: $^1/_{1000} \times 60 = ^3/_{50}$

   $^1/_{100} \times 6 = ^3/_{50}$

4. $\frac{1}{4}:500::x:1000$

$500x = \frac{1}{4} \times 1000$

$500x = \frac{1}{4} \times \frac{1000}{1} = 250$

$\frac{\cancel{500}x}{\cancel{500}} = \frac{250}{500} = 250 \div 500 = 0.5$

$x = 0.5$

$500 \times 0.5 = 250$
$\frac{1}{4} \times 1000 = 250$

5. $36:12::\frac{1}{100}:x$

$36x = 12 \times \frac{1}{100}$

$36x = \frac{12}{1} \times \frac{1}{100} = \frac{3}{25}$

$\frac{\cancel{36}x}{\cancel{36}} = \frac{3/25}{36} = \frac{3}{25} \div 36 = \frac{3}{25} \times \frac{1}{36} = \frac{1}{300}$

$x = \frac{1}{300}$

$36 \times \frac{1}{300} = \frac{3}{25}$
$12 \times \frac{1}{100} = \frac{3}{25}$

6. $6:24::0.75:x$

$6x = 24 \times 0.75 = 18$
$6x = 18$

$\frac{\cancel{6}x}{\cancel{6}} = \frac{18}{6} = 18 \div 6 = 3$

$x = 3$

$24 \times 0.75 = 18$
$6 \times 3 = 18$

7. $x:600::4:120$

$120x = 4 \times 600 = 2400$

$\frac{\cancel{120}x}{\cancel{120}} = \frac{2400}{120} = 2400 \div 120 = 20$

$x = 20$

$600 \times 4 = 2400$
$20 \times 120 = 2400$

8. $0.7:70::x:1000$

$70x = 0.7 \times 1000 = 700$

$\frac{\cancel{70}x}{\cancel{70}} = \frac{700}{70} = 700 \div 70 = 10$

$x = 10$

$70 \times 10 = 700$
$0.7 \times 1000 = 700$

9. $9:27::300:x$

$9x = 27 \times 300 = 8100$

$$\frac{\cancel{9}x}{\cancel{9}} = \frac{8100}{9} = 8100 \div 9 = 900$$

$x = 900$

PROOF: $27 \times 300 = 8100$

$9 \times 900 = 8100$

10. $6:12::\frac{1}{4}:x$

$6x = 12 \times \frac{1}{4} = 3$

$$\frac{\cancel{6}x}{\cancel{6}} = \frac{3}{6} = 3 \div 6 = 0.5$$

$x = 0.5$

PROOF: $12 \times \frac{1}{4} = 3$

$6 \times 0.5 = 3$

2C Answer sheet

1. $\frac{1}{200}:x::1:800$

$1x = \frac{1}{200} \times 800$

$$1x = \frac{1}{200} \times \frac{800}{1} = 4$$

$$\frac{\cancel{1}x}{\cancel{1}} = \frac{4}{1} = 4 \div 1 = 4$$

$x = 4$

PROOF: $4 \times 1 = 4$

$\frac{1}{200} \times 800 = 4$

2. $15:30::x:12$

$30x = 15 \times 12$

$30x = 180$

$$\frac{\cancel{30}x}{\cancel{30}} = \frac{180}{30} = 180 \div 30 = 6$$

$x = 6$

PROOF: $30 \times 6 = 180$

$15 \times 12 = 180$

3. $\frac{1}{1000}:\frac{1}{100}::x:30$

$\frac{1}{100}x = \frac{1}{1000} \times 30$

$$\frac{1}{100}x = \frac{1}{1000} \times \frac{30}{1} = \frac{3}{100}$$

$$\frac{\cancel{\frac{1}{100}}x}{\cancel{\frac{1}{100}}} = \frac{\frac{3}{100}}{\frac{1}{100}} = \frac{3}{100} \div \frac{1}{100} = \frac{3}{100} \times \frac{100}{1} = 3$$

$x = 3$

PROOF: $\frac{1}{1000} \times 30 = \frac{3}{100}$

$\frac{1}{100} \times 3 = \frac{3}{100}$

4. $6:12::0.25:x$

$6x = 12 \times 0.25 = 3$

$\dfrac{\cancel{6}x}{\cancel{6}} = \dfrac{3}{6} = 3 \div 6 = 0.5$

$x = 0.5$

5. $300:5::x:{}^1\!/_{60}$

$5x = {}^1\!/_{60} \times 300$

$5x = \dfrac{1}{60} \times \dfrac{300}{1} = 5$

$\dfrac{\cancel{5}x}{5} = \dfrac{5}{5} = 5 \div 5 = 1$

$x = 1$

6. ${}^1\!/_{150}:{}^1\!/_{200}::2:x$

${}^1\!/_{150}x = {}^1\!/_{200} \times 2$

$\dfrac{1}{150}x = \dfrac{1}{200} \times \dfrac{2}{1} = \dfrac{1}{100}$

$\dfrac{{}^{\cancel{1}}\!/_{\cancel{150}}x}{{}^{\cancel{1}}\!/_{\cancel{150}}} = \dfrac{{}^1\!/_{100}}{{}^1\!/_{150}} = \dfrac{1}{100} \div \dfrac{1}{150} = \dfrac{1}{100} \times \dfrac{150}{1} = \dfrac{3}{2} = 1{}^1\!/_2$

$x = 1{}^1\!/_2$

7. ${}^1\!/_2:{}^1\!/_6::{}^1\!/_4:x$

${}^1\!/_2x = {}^1\!/_6 \times {}^1\!/_4 = {}^1\!/_{24}$

$\dfrac{{}^{\cancel{1}}\!/_{\cancel{2}}x}{{}^{\cancel{1}}\!/_{\cancel{2}}} = \dfrac{{}^1\!/_{24}}{{}^1\!/_2} = \dfrac{1}{24} \div \dfrac{1}{2} = \dfrac{1}{24} \times \dfrac{2}{1} = \dfrac{1}{12}$

$x = {}^1\!/_{12}$

8. $7.5:12::x:28$

$12x = 7.5 \times 28 = 210$

$\dfrac{\cancel{12}x}{\cancel{12}} = \dfrac{210}{12} = 210 \div 12 = 17.5$

$x = 17.5$

9. $15:x::1.5:10$

$1.5x = 15 \times 10 = 150$

$\dfrac{\cancel{1.5}x}{\cancel{1.5}} = \dfrac{150}{1.5} = 150 \div 1.5 = 100$

$x = 100$

PROOF: $15 \times 10 = 150$

$100 \times 1.5 = 150$

2D Answer sheet

1. **Have**   **Want to know**

Scoops : Cups : : Scoops : Cups

$4:6::x:18$

$6x = 72$

$\dfrac{\cancel{6}x}{\cancel{6}} = \dfrac{72}{6} = 12$

$x = 12$ scoops of cocoa

PROOF: $4:6::12:18$

$6 \times 12 = 72$

$4 \times 18 = 72$

REMEMBER: Scoops : Cups : : Scoops : Cups

Apples : Bananas : : Apples : Bananas

Miles : Gallons : : Miles : Gallons

You want x to stand alone. To get x to stand alone, divide by 6. Whatever you do on one side of an equation, you must do on the other.

Obtain proof by putting your answer back into the equation in place of x. Multiply the two inside numbers, and they should equal the two outside numbers.

2. **Have**   **Want to know**

Scoops : Cups : : Scoops : Cups

$7:8::x:40$

$8x = 40 \times 7 = 280$

$\dfrac{\cancel{8}x}{\cancel{8}} = \dfrac{280}{8} = 35$

$x = 35$ scoops

PROOF: $7:8::35:40$

$8 \times 35 = 280$

$7 \times 40 = 280$

3. **Have**   **Want to know**

Bananas : Apples : : Bananas : Apples

$6 : 9 : : x : 72$

$9x = 6 \times 72 = 432$

$\dfrac{\cancel{9}x}{\cancel{9}} = \dfrac{432}{9} = 48$

$x = 48$ bananas

4. **Have**   **Want to know**

300 mg : 1 tab. : : 450 mg : x tab.

$300x = 450$

$\dfrac{\cancel{300}x}{\cancel{300}} = \dfrac{450}{300} = 1.5$

$x = 1.5$ tablets

Always label your answer.

PROOF: $300 : 1 : : 450 : 1.5$

$1 \times 450 = 450$

$300 \times 1.5 = 450$

5. **Have**   **Want to know**

Bushes : Trees : : Bushes : Trees

$8 : 2 : : x : 36$

$2x = 8 \times 36 = 288$

$\dfrac{\cancel{2}x}{\cancel{2}} = \dfrac{288}{2} = 144$

$x = 144$ bushes

PROOF: $8 : 2 : : 144 : 36$

$8 \times 36 = 288$

$2 \times 144 = 288$

6. **Have**   **Want to know**

Cups : Day : : Cups : Day

$4 : 1 : : 84 : x$

$4x = 84$

$\dfrac{\cancel{4}x}{\cancel{4}} = \dfrac{84}{4} = 21$

$x = 21$ days

PROOF: $4 : 1 : : 84 : 21$

$1 \times 84 = 84$

$4 \times 21 = 84$

7. **Have**   **Want to know**

Cups : Loaves : : Cups : Loaves

$4 : 3 : : 24 : x$

$4x = 72$

$\dfrac{\cancel{4}x}{\cancel{4}} = \dfrac{72}{4} = 18$

$x = 18$ loaves

PROOF: $4 : 3 : : 24 : 18$

$4 \times 18 = 72$

$3 \times 24 = 72$

2E Answer sheet

1. **Have**   **Need**

   $5 \text{ mg} : 1 \text{ tab.} :: 40 \text{ mg} : x \text{ tab.}$

   $5x = 40$

   $x = 8 \text{ tablets}$

   PROOF: $40 \times 1 = 40$
$5 \times 8 = 40$

2. a. More: $\frac{1}{4}$ is more than $\frac{1}{6}$.

   b. $\frac{1}{6} \text{ gr} : 1 \text{ tab.} :: \frac{1}{4} \text{ gr} : x \text{ tab.}$

   $\frac{1}{6}x = \frac{1}{4}$

   To get x to stand alone, divide the number by itself:

   $$\frac{\frac{1}{6}x}{\frac{1}{6}} = \frac{\cancel{\frac{1}{6}}x}{\cancel{\frac{1}{6}}} = x$$

   What you do to one side you must do to the other side of the equation. Now put $\frac{1}{6}$ under $\frac{1}{4}$. This means:

   $$x = \frac{\frac{1}{4}}{\frac{1}{6}} \text{ or } \frac{1}{4} \div \frac{1}{6}$$

   PROOF: $\frac{1}{6} \times 1\frac{1}{2} = \frac{1}{4}$

   $1 \times \frac{1}{4} = \frac{1}{4}$

   The problem now looks like this:

   $$\frac{\cancel{\frac{1}{6}}x}{\cancel{\frac{1}{6}}} = \frac{\frac{1}{4}}{\frac{1}{6}} = \frac{1}{4} \div \frac{1}{6} = \frac{1}{4} \times \frac{6}{1} = \frac{3}{2} = 1\frac{1}{2}$$

   $x = 1\frac{1}{2} \text{ tablets}$

3. $\frac{1}{8} \text{ gr} : 1 \text{ tab.} :: \frac{1}{6} \text{ gr} : x \text{ tab.}$

   a. More: $\frac{1}{6}$ is more than $\frac{1}{8}$.

   b. $\frac{1}{8}x = \frac{1}{6}$

   PROOF: $\frac{1}{8} \times 1\frac{1}{3} = \frac{1}{6}$

   $1 \times \frac{1}{6} = \frac{1}{6}$

   $$\frac{\cancel{\frac{1}{8}}x}{\cancel{\frac{1}{8}}} = \frac{\frac{1}{6}}{\frac{1}{8}} = \frac{1}{6} \div \frac{1}{8} = \frac{1}{6} \times \frac{8}{1} = 1\frac{1}{3}$$

   $x = 1\frac{1}{3} \text{ tablets}$

4. $3 \text{ water} : 2 \text{ apples} :: 24 \text{ water} : x \text{ apples}$

   $3x = 48$

   PROOF: $3 : 2 :: 24 : 16$

   $3 \times 16 = 48$

   $2 \times 24 = 48$

   $$\frac{\cancel{3}x}{\cancel{3}} = \frac{48}{3} = 16$$

   $x = 16 \text{ apples}$

5. 6 pens : 8 pencils : : x pens : 72 pencils
   $8x = 432$

   $$\frac{\cancel{8}x}{\cancel{8}} = \frac{432}{8} = 54$$

   $x = 54$ pens

   PROOF: $6 : 8 : : 54 : 72$
   $6 \times 72 = 432$
   $8 \times 54 = 432$

6. ½ tsp. salt : 3 eggs : : x tsp. salt : 30 eggs
   $3x = 30 \times ½$

   $$3x = \frac{30}{1} \times \frac{1}{2} = \frac{30}{2} = 15$$

   $$\frac{\cancel{3}x}{\cancel{3}} = \frac{15}{3} = 5$$

   $x = 5$ tsp. salt

   PROOF: $½ : 3 : : 5 : 30$
   $3 \times 5 = 15$
   $½ \times 30 = 15$

7. 8 cups : 7 scoops : : 24 cups : x scoops
   $8x = 7 \times 24$

   $$\frac{\cancel{8}x}{\cancel{8}} = \frac{168}{8} = 21$$

   $x = 21$ scoops

   PROOF: $8 : 7 : : 24 : 21$
   $8 \times 21 = 168$
   $7 \times 24 = 168$

Section 2 RATIO AND PROPORTION QUIZ

SHOW ALL WORK.

Solve the following proportions for x:

1. $9:x::5:300$

2. $6:24::0.75:x$

3. $8:16::x:24$

4. $x:600::4:120$

5. $5:3000::15:x$

6. $0.7:70::x:1000$

7. $9:27::300:x$

8. $6:12::\frac{1}{4}:x$

9. $25:x::75:3000$

10. $0.6:10::0.5:x$

Section 2 Ratio and proportion quiz answer sheet _____

1. 540
2. 3
3. 12
4. 20

5. 9000
6. 10
7. 900

8. 0.5 or $\frac{1}{2}$
9. 1000
10. $8\frac{1}{3}$

SECTION 3

Metric system

UNIT A_____

Math objectives

1. *Memorize milligram, gram, and kilogram conversions.*
2. *Memorize milliliter and liter conversions.*

Explanation

The metric system is now being used exclusively in the United States Pharmacopeia and before long will probably be the only system used in drug dosage. Arabic numbers and decimals are used with this system. Blame the French if you don't like the metric system, but it's really easier than any other method because it is a decimal system (based on the number 10) and all the math involved is done by moving decimals.

The basic metric units are multiplied and divided always by a multiple of *10* to form the entire system. (The period for abbreviation often may not appear in some writings.) There are only a few equivalents that are used in medicine. These are as follows:

MEMORIZE:

Weight

1 mg (milligram)   = 1000 μg (or mcg) (micrograms)
1 g (gram)   = 1000 mg (milligrams)
1 kg (kilogram) = 2.2 lb = 1000 g or Gm (grams)

Volume

1000 ml (milliliters) or cc (cubic centimeters) = 1 L (liter)

A milliliter (ml) is equivalent to a cubic centimeter (cc) and for all practical purposes these units may be used interchangeably. However, the use of milliliter is preferable. Hence:

$$1000 \text{ cc} = 1 \text{ L (liter)}$$
$$1000 \text{ ml} = 1 \text{ L (liter)}$$

Section 3 answer sheets begin on p. 64.

PLEASE NOTE: The symbol, such as g or mg, always *follows* the amount.

EXAMPLE: 1000 mg
              1 g

NOTE: Some doctors may use the symbol mgm for mg (milligram) and Gm for g (gram). The symbol mcg is becoming obsolete.

Metric measurements, prefixes, and their equivalents

Prefix	Numerical value	Power of base 10	Meaning
giga	1,000,000,000.	10^9	One billion times
mega	1,000,000.	10^6	One million times
*kilo	1,000.	10^3	One thousand times
hecto	100.	10^2	One hundred times
deka	10.	10^1	Ten times
deci	.1	10^{-1}	Tenth part of
*centi	.01	10^{-2}	Hundredth part of
*milli	.001	10^{-3}	Thousandth part of
*micro	.000001	10^{-6}	Millionth part of
*nano	.000000001	10^{-9}	Billionth part of

These prefixes can be combined with liters and grams.

	Weight	Volume
EXAMPLE:	decigram (dg)	deciliter (dl)
	dekagram (dkg)	dekaliter (dkl)
	hectogram (hg)	hectaliter (hl)
	centigram (cg)	centiliter (cl)
	kilogram (kg)	kiloliter (kl)
	milligram (mg)	milliliter (ml)

---

*Prefixes most frequently used in computing dosages.

UNIT B

Math objective

Calculate gram and milligram conversion problems.

Conversions

<small>REMEMBER:</small> 1 g = 1000 mg

The metric system is a decimal system. To convert g (large) to mg (small), multiply by 1000 or move the decimal point 3 places to the right (for *1000* times smaller).

To convert mg (small) to g (large), divide by *1000* or move the decimal point 3 places to the left (for *1000* times greater).

<small>**EXAMPLE:**</small>   We know 1000 mg = 1 g

Therefore 1500 mg = 1.5 g   ·

Divide 1500 mg by 1000 × 1.5 g, or move decimal 3 places to the left for converting mg (small) to g (large).

Therefore 5 g = 5000 mg

Multiply 5 g by 1000 = 5000 mg, or move decimal 3 places to the right for converting g (large) to mg (small).

3B Worksheet

<small>REMEMBER:</small> 1 g = 1000 mg

1. 1 g = _____ mg

2. 2 g = _____ mg

3. 1.5 g = _____ mg

4. 0.5 g = _____ mg

5. ½ g = _____ mg

6. 0.25 g = _____ mg

7. 0.05 g = _____ mg

8. 0.1 g = _____ mg

9. 1.1 g = _____ mg

10. 0.3 g = _____ mg

11. 25 mg = _____ g

12. 5 mg = _____ g

13. 3000 mg = _____ g

14. 1500 mg = _____ g

15. 15,000 mg = _____ g

16. 10 mg = _____ g

17. 100 mg = _____ g

18. 0.5 mg = _____ g

19. 7.5 mg = _____ g

UNIT C

Math objective

Calculate one-step metric conversion problems by ratio and proportion method.

Ratio and proportion

RULE: **1** To solve metric problems, first analyze the problem.

EXAMPLE: 40 mg = _____ g

You already know you can move the decimal point 3 places to the left (divide) and come out with the correct answer. However, now it's time to start setting up a ratio and proportion problem.

1 What we *know* goes on the *left*.

2 What we *want to know* (the x, or unknown) goes on the *right*.

Know	Want to know

$1 \text{ g} : 1000 \text{ mg} :: x \text{ g} : 40 \text{ mg}$ PROOF: $1000 \times 0.04 = 40$

$1000x = 40$ $1 \times 40 = 40$

$$\frac{\cancel{1000}x}{\cancel{1000}} = \frac{40}{1000} = 40 \div 1000$$

$$\begin{array}{r} .04 \\ 1000\overline{)40.00} \\ \underline{40\ 00} \end{array}$$

$x = 0.04$ g   Always *label* your answer.

3C Worksheet _____

Show all work, prove, and label all answers:

REMEMBER: 1 mg = 1000 μg
  1 g = 1000 mg
  1 kg (2.2 lb) = 1000 g
  1 L = 1000 ml

Use ratio and proportion:

1. 25 mg = _____ g

2. 0.064 g = _____ mg

3. 4 mg = _____ g

4. 4.6 g = _____ mg

5. 375 ml = _____ L

6. 89 kg = _____ g

7. 45 mg = _____ g

8. 0.6 g = _____ mg

9. 50 kg = _____ lb

UNIT D

Math objectives

1. *Identify one- and two-step metric conversion problems.*
2. *Calculate two-step metric conversion problems by ratio and proportion method.*

Two-step problems

MUST KNOW

$1000\ \mu g = 1\ mg$

$1000\ mg = 1\ g$

$1000\ g = 1\ kg$

$1000\ ml = 1\ L$

Two-step ratio and proportion

EXAMPLE: The doctor ordered 10 mg. On hand you have 0.002 g each tablet. How many tablets will you give?

Step 1: Have g on hand. Need to change mg to g because that is what is on hand. What do you know about g and mg?

Know   Want to know

1000 mg : 1 g : : 10 mg : x g   PROOF: $1000 \times 0.01 = 10$

*Cancel x out: $1 \times 10 = 10$

$$\frac{\cancel{1000}x}{\cancel{1000}} = \frac{10}{1000} = 10 \div 1000 = 0.01$$

$x = 0.01$ g

The doctor ordered 10 mg. We now know that 10 mg = 0.01 g. Now set up the second step to solve the problem.

Step 2: Know   Want to know

0.002 g : 1 tab. : : 0.01 g : x tab.   PROOF: $0.002 \times 5 = 0.01$

*Cancel x out: $1 \times 0.01 = 0.01$

$$\frac{\cancel{0.002}x}{\cancel{0.002}} = \frac{0.01}{0.002} = 0.01 \div 0.002 = 5$$

$x = 5$ tablets of 0.002 g each

---

*There is no need to cancel out if you make sure to put the x on the *left* side and remember to divide the x into the sum on the *right* side of the equation.

3D Worksheet _____

Two-step metric problems. Show all work, set up ratio and proportion, prove, and label all work. Remember to estimate your answer when you reach the second step.

1. Doctor ordered 0.75 g of erythromycin. On hand you have 250 mg tablets. How many tablets will you give?

$$.75g \times \frac{1000mg}{1g} \times \frac{Tab}{250} =$$

3

2. Doctor ordered Valium 10 mg. On hand you have Valium 0.005 g tablets. How many tablets will you give?

3. Ordered are 3 mg of codeine. On hand you have 0.002 g tablets of codeine. How many tablets will you give?

4. Doctor ordered 75 mg of Demerol IM. On hand you have a vial of 0.050 g per ml. How many ml will you give?

5. Doctor ordered chlorpromazine 0.075 g. On hand you have chlorpromazine 25 mg/ml. How many ml will you give?

6. Ordered are 2 g of Staphcillin. The vial reads: ''Add 8.6 ml of diluent to contents of vial. Each ml will contain 500 mg of Staphcillin.'' You will administer how many ml?

7. Doctor ordered 500 mg of Gantrisin. Available is Gantrisin 0.25 g tablets. How many tablets will you give?

8. You are to give 0.125 g of Keflin. On hand you have Keflin 50 mg/5 ml. How many ml will you give? The Keflin will be administered in an intravenous solution.

Section 3 METRIC SYSTEM ANSWER SHEETS

3B Answer sheet

1. 1000 mg
2. 2000 mg
3. 1500 mg
4. 500 mg
5. 500 mg
6. 250 mg
7. 50 mg

8. 100 mg
9. 1100 mg
10. 300 mg
11. 0.025 g
12. 0.005 g
13. 3 g

14. 1.5 g
15. 15 g
16. 0.010 g
17. 0.100 g
18. 0.0005 g
19. 0.0075 g

3C Answer sheet

1. **Know**   **Want to know**

   1000 mg : 1 g :: 25 mg : x g

   $$\frac{\cancel{1000}x}{\cancel{1000}} = \frac{25}{1000} = 25 \div 1000$$

   $x = 0.025$ g

   PROOF: $1000 \times 0.025 = 25$
   $1 \times 25 = 25$

2. **Know**   **Want to know**

   1000 mg : 1 g :: x mg : 0.064 g
   $1x = 1000 \times 0.064$
   $x = 64$ mg

   PROOF: $1 \times 64 = 64$
   $1000 \times 0.064 = 64$

3. **Know**   **Want to know**

   1000 mg : 1 g :: 4 mg : x g
   $1000x = 4$

   $$\frac{\cancel{1000}x}{\cancel{1000}} = \frac{4}{1000} = 4 \div 1000$$

   $x = 0.004$ g

   PROOF: $1000 \times 0.004 = 4$
   $1 \times 4 = 4$

4. **Know**   **Want to know**

   1000 mg : 1 g :: x mg : 4.6 g
   $1x = 1000 \times 4.6$
   $x = 4600$ mg

   PROOF: $1 \times 4600 = 4600$
   $1000 \times 4.6 = 4600$

5. **Know**   **Want to know**

    1000 ml:1 L::375 ml:x L

    $1000x = 375$

    $$\frac{\cancel{1000}x}{\cancel{1000}} = \frac{375}{1000} = 375 \div 1000$$

    $x = 0.375$ L

    PROOF: $0.375 \times 1000 = 375$
    $1 \times 375 = 375$

6. **Know**   **Want to know**

    1000 g:1 kg::x g:89 kg

    $1x = 89,000$

    $x = 89,000$ g

    PROOF: $1 \times 89,000 = 89,000$
    $1000 \times 89 = 89,000$

7. **Know**   **Want to know**

    1000 mg:1 g::45 mg:x g

    $1000x = 45$

    $$\frac{\cancel{1000}x}{\cancel{1000}} = \frac{45}{1000} = 45 \div 1000$$

    $x = 0.045$ g

    PROOF: $1000 \times 0.045 = 45$
    $1 \times 45 = 45$

8. **Know**   **Want to know**

    1000 mg:1 g::x mg:0.6 g

    $1x = 1000 \times 0.6$

    $x = 600$ mg

    PROOF: $1 \times 600 = 600$
    $1000 \times 0.6 = 600$

9. **Know**   **Want to know**

    1 kg:2.2 lb::50 kg:x lb

    $1x = 50 \times 2.2$

    $x = 110$ lb

    PROOF: $2.2 \times 50 = 110$
    $1 \times 110 = 110$

3D Answer sheet

1. *Step 1:*

   Know   **Want to know**

   1000 mg : 1 g : : x mg : 0.75 g

   $1x = 750$

   $x = 750$ mg

   PROOF: $1000 \times 0.75 = 750$

   $1 \times 750 = 750$

   Must change g into mg because that is what is available.

   Step 2:

   Know or have   **Want to know**

   250 mg : 1 tab. : : 750 mg : x tab.

   $$\frac{250x}{250} = \frac{750}{250} = 750 \div 250$$

   $x = 3$ tablets

   PROOF: $250 \times 3 = 750$

   $1 \times 750 = 750$

   You must give 3 tablets of 250 mg each to give required amount of 750 mg.

2. *Step 1:*

   Know   **Want to know**

   1000 mg : 1 g : : 10 mg : x g

   $1000x = 10$

   $x = 0.01$ g

   PROOF: $1000 \times 0.01 = 10$

   $1 \times 10 = 10$

   Step 2:

   Know or have   **Want to know**

   0.005 g : 1 tab. : : 0.01 g : x tab.

   $$\frac{0.005x}{0.005} = \frac{0.01}{0.005}$$

   $x = 2$ tablets of 0.005 g

   PROOF: $1 \times 0.01 = 0.01$

   $0.005 \times 2 = 0.01$

3. *Step 1:*

   Know   **Want to know**

   1000 mg : 1 g : : 3 mg : x g

   $1000x = 3$

   $x = 0.003$ g

   PROOF: $1 \times 3 = 3$

   $1000 \times 0.003 = 3$

Step 2:

Know or have   **Want to know**

0.002 g:1 tab.::0.003 g:x tab.

0.002x = 0.003

x = 1.5 tablets

PROOF: 1 × 0.003 = 0.003

         0.002 × 1.5 = 0.003

You will give 1½ tablets of 0.002 g.

4. *Step 1:*

Know   **Want to know**

1000 mg:1 g::75 mg:x g

1000x = 75

x = 0.075 g

PROOF: 1 × 75 = 75

         1000 × 0.075 = 75

Step 2:

Know or have   **Want to know**

0.050 g:1 ml::0.075 g:x ml

0.050x = 0.075

x = 1.5 ml or 1½ ml

PROOF: 1 × 0.075 = 0.075

         0.050× 1.5 = 0.075

5. *Step 1:*

Know   **Want to know**

1000 mg:1 g::x mg:0.075 g

1x = 75 mg

x = 75 mg

PROOF: 1 × 75 = 75

         1000 × 0.075 = 75

Step 2:

Know or have   **Want to know**

25 mg:1 ml::75 mg:x ml

25x = 75

x = 3 ml

PROOF: 1 × 75 = 75

         25 × 3 = 75

6. *Step 1:*

Know   **Want to know**

1000 mg:1 g::x mg:2 g

1x = 2000

x = 2000 mg

PROOF: 1 × 2000 = 2000

         1000 × 2 = 2000

Step 2:

Know or have   **Want to know**

500 mg:1 ml::2000 mg:x ml

500x = 2000

x = 4 ml

PROOF: 1 × 2000 = 2000

500 × 4 = 2000

7. *Step 1:*

Know   **Want to know**

1000 mg:1 g::500 mg:x g

1000x = 500

x = 0.5 g

PROOF: 1 × 500 = 500

1000 × 0.5 = 500

Step 2:

Know or have   **Want to know**

0.25 g:1 tab.::0.5 g:x tab.

0.25x = 0.5

x = 2 tablets

PROOF: 1 × 0.5 = 0.5

0.25 × 2 = 0.5

8. *Step 1:*

Know   **Want to know**

1000 mg:1 g::x mg:0.125 g

1x = 125

x = 125 mg

PROOF: 1000 × 0.125 = 125

1 × 125 = 125

Step 2:

Know or have **Want to know**

50 mg:5 ml::125 mg:x ml

50x = 625

x = 12.5 ml of Keflin IV

PROOF: 50 × 12.5 = 625

5 × 125 = 625

Section 3 METRIC QUIZ

Use ratio and proportion. Estimate your answer; label and prove answer.

1. 500 mg = _____ g

2. 25 mg = _____ g

3. 5 mg = _____ g

4. 2500 mg = _____ g

5. 12 mg = _____ g

6. 4 g = _____ mg

7. 65 mg = _____ g

8. Doctor ordered 10 mg of Valium. On hand you have 0.02 g in each tablet. How many tablets will you give? (Is this a one-step or a two-step problem?) Prove.

9. Doctor ordered 60 mg. On hand you have 20 mg tablets. How many tablets will you give? (Is this a one-step or a two-step problem?)

10. Ordered is 0.75 g. On hand you have 250 mg tablets. How many tablets will you give? (Is this a one-step or two-step problem?)

11. Doctor ordered 500 mg of Achromycin. On hand are 250 mg tablets. You will give _____ tablets.

12. Digitoxin 0.125 mg tablets are on hand. Give 0.25 mg. How many tablets will you give?

Section 3 Metric quiz answer sheet

1. 0.5 g
2. 0.025 g
3. 0.005 g
4. 2.5 g
5. 0.012 g
6. 4000 mg

7. 0.065 g
8. ½ tablet (two-step problem)
9. 3 tablets (one-step problem)
10. 3 tablets (two-step problem)
11. 2 tablets
12. 2 tablets

SECTION 4

Apothecary system

UNIT A

Math objective

Memorize symbols for dram, ounce, drop, and minim.

Apothecary measures

VOLUME (WET)

gtt = drop = minim (℔, ℔, or m.)
60 minims (℔) = 1 dram (dr or ʒ) = 1 tsp. = 5 ml = 60 gtt
8 dr (ʒ) = 1 ounce (oz or ℥) = 30 ml = 8 tsp.
16 oz (℥) = 1 pint (pt or O.) = 500 ml
2 pt = 1 quart (qt) = 1000 ml
4 qt = 1 gallon (gal or C) = 4000 ml
480 ℔ = 1 oz (℥) = 30 ml
32 oz (℥) = 1 qt = 1000 ml

MUST KNOW:

ʒ = dram (dr)

℥ = ounce (oz)

gtt = drop

℔ = minim

Section 4 answer sheets begin on p. 78.

UNIT B

Equivalents

Table 1. Approximate equivalents of metric, apothecary, and household measures

Household	Apothecary	Metric
60 drops (gtt)	1 teaspoon (tsp.)	5 ml (or cc)*
1 drop (gtt)	1 minim	0.065 g
	15 or 16 minims	1 ml
1 teaspoon (tsp.)	1 fluidram	5 ml
1 tablespoon (tbs.)	4 fluidrams	15 ml
2 tablespoons (tbs.)	8 fluidrams	30 ml
1 cup	4 or 5 ounces	120-150 ml
1 glass	5 or 6 ounces	150-180 ml
1 pint bottle	1 pint or 16 ounces	500 ml
1 quart bottle	1 quart or 32 ounces	1000 ml

*The abbreviations *ml* and *cc* are used interchangeably; however, *ml* should be used for liquids, *cc* for solids and gases, and *g* for solids.

Math objective

Read roman numerals.

Roman numerals and Arabic numerals

Roman numerals are used with the apothecary system. Usually Arabic numerals are used for numbers over 9. Fractions are written with Arabic numerals except for $\overline{ss}$ (semis), which stands for one half. If the quantity is composed of a whole number and a fraction, the entire amount is written in Arabic numerals.

Arabic numerals	Capital roman numerals	Small roman numerals
1	I	i
2	II	ii
3	III	iii
4	IV	iv
5	V	v
6	VI	vi
7	VII	vii
8	VIII	viii
9	IX	ix
10	X	x
19	XIX	xix
20	XX	xx
30	XXX	xxx
40	XL	xl
49	XLIX	xlix
50	L	l
60	LX	lx
70	LXX	lxx
80	LXXX	lxxx
90	XC	xc
100	C	c
500	D	d
1000	M	m

In the apothecary system the measure or symbol precedes the number.

EXAMPLE: gr xv, gr XV

ʒ i (in handwriting: ʒ i̇)

ʒ ii (in handwriting: ʒ i̇i̇)

gr $\overline{ss}$ (one half)

gtt ii (drops)

UNIT C

Math objective

Calculate one-step apothecary system problems.

Ratio and proportion

EXAMPLE: You have a vial of caffeine containing gr 1½ per ml. Doctor ordered caffeine gr 3¾. How many ml will you give?

What was ordered and what you *have* on hand are in the same system; therefore it is a one-step problem.

REMEMBER: *Have* or *know* goes on the *left*.

Have   **Want to know**

gr 1½ : 1 ml :: gr 3¾ : x ml

$$\frac{\cancel{1\frac{1}{2}}x}{\cancel{1\frac{1}{2}}} = \frac{3\frac{3}{4}}{1\frac{1}{2}} = \frac{15}{4} \div \frac{3}{2} = \frac{15}{4} \times \frac{2}{3} = \frac{30}{12} = 2\frac{1}{2}$$

$x = 2\frac{1}{2}$ ml = 2.5 ml

PROOF: $1 \times 3\frac{3}{4} = 3\frac{3}{4}$

$1\frac{1}{2} \times 2\frac{1}{2} = 3\frac{3}{4}$

4C Worksheet

Using ratio and proportion, prove:

1. You are to give codeine gr i. You have codeine gr $\overline{ss}$ per ml. How many ml will you give?

2. You are to give ASA gr XV. You have ASA gr V per tablet. How many tablets will you give?

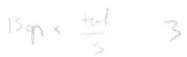

3. Doctor ordered M.S. gr ⅙. You have on hand a vial containing M.S. gr ⅛ per ml. How many ml will you give? (For amounts over 1 ml, calculate to tenths; for amounts under 1 ml, calculate to hundredths.)

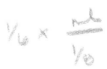

4. Doctor ordered an aminophylline suppository gr XV. On hand you have aminophylline suppository gr viiss. How many suppositories will you give?

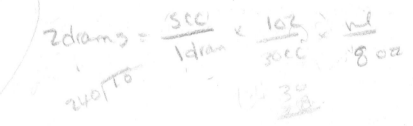

5. On hand you have a can of Metamucil containing ʒ viii. You are to give Metamucil ʒ ii. How many tsp. will you mix with juice or water? How many ml is this?

6. You are to give ʒ ss of Maalox. On hand you have a bottle containing Maalox ʒ viii. How many ml will you give?

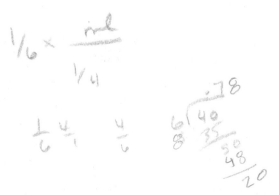

7. You are to give codeine gr ⅙ SC. On hand you have codeine gr ¼ per ml. How many ml will you give? Your immediate reaction will be to give _____ (more or less) than 1 ml. (Calculate to hundredths. Do not round.)

UNIT D

Math objective

Calculate one-step and two-step apothecary system problems.

4D Worksheet

1. Doctor ordered M.S. (morphine sulfate) gr $^1/_8$. On hand you have a vial containing M.S. gr $^1/_{10}$ per ml. How many minims will you give?

2. Doctor ordered Robitussin ℥ $^1/_4$. How many drams (ʒ) will you give?

3. Doctor ordered atropine gr $^1/_{200}$. On hand you have an ampule of atropine labeled gr $^1/_{150}$ per 0.5 ml. How many ml. will you give? How many minims will you give?

4. On hand you have Gantrisin tablets gr V. Doctor ordered Gantrisin tablets gr 15. How many tablets will you give?

5. Doctor ordered ℥ $\overline{ss}$ of cough syrup. How many drams is this? How many ml will you give?

77

Section 4 APOTHECARY SYSTEM ANSWER SHEETS

4C Answer sheet

REMEMBER: *Have* or *know* goes on the left.

1. **Have**   **Want to know**

   gr $^1/_2 : 1$ ml $:: $ gr $1 : x$ ml

   $$\frac{\cancel{^1/_2}x}{\cancel{^1/_2}} = \frac{1}{^1/_2} = 1 \div ^1/_2 = 1 \times 2 = 2$$

   $x = 2$ ml

   PROOF: $^1/_2 \times 2 = 1$
   $1 \times 1 = 1$

2. **Have**   **Want to know**

   gr $5 : 1$ tab. $::$ gr $15 : x$ tab.
   $5x = 15$
   $x = 3$ tablets

   PROOF: $5 \times 3 = 15$
   $1 \times 15 = 15$

3. **Have**   **Want to know**

   gr $^1/_8 : 1$ ml $::$ gr $^1/_6 : x$ ml

   $$\frac{\cancel{^1/_8}x}{\cancel{^1/_8}} = \frac{^1/_6}{^1/_8} = \frac{1}{6} \div \frac{1}{8} = \frac{1}{6} \times \frac{8}{1} = \frac{4}{3} = 1^1/_3$$

   $x = 1^1/_3$ ml

   PROOF: $^1/_8 \times 1^1/_3 = ^1/_6$
   $1 \times ^1/_6 = ^1/_6$

   Answer must be a decimal. Therefore: $1^1/_3 = ^4/_3 = $

   $$
   \begin{array}{r}
   1.33 = 1.33 \\
   3\overline{)4.00} \\
   \underline{3} \\
   1\,0 \\
   \underline{9} \\
   10 \\
   \underline{9} \\
   1
   \end{array}
   $$

   Give 1.3 ml of morphine sulfate.

4. **Have**   **Want to know**

gr 7.5:1 supp. :: gr 15:x supp.

PROOF: $7.5 \times 2 = 15$
$1 \times 15 = 15$

$$\frac{\cancel{7}x}{\cancel{7}} = \frac{15}{7} = 15 \div 7 = \frac{15}{1} \times \frac{1}{7} = \frac{15}{7} = 2\frac{1}{7}$$

$x = 2$ suppositories

Give 2 suppositories.

5. This is a two-step problem. You must find out what part ʒ i (dr) is to ʒ i (oz).

Know   **Want to know**

ʒ ï:1 tsp. :: ʒ ïï:x tsp.

$x = 1 \times 2 = 2$

$x = 2$ tsp.

PROOF: $1 \times 2 = 2$
$1 \times 2 = 2$

Know   **Want to know**

1 tsp.:5 ml::2 tsp.:x ml

$x = 5 \times 2 = 10$

$x = 10$ ml

PROOF: $1 \times 10 = 10$
$5 \times 2 = 10$

6. What do you know about ʒ and ml?

Know   **Want to know**

30 ml:1 oz::x ml:$\frac{1}{2}$ oz

PROOF: $30 \times \frac{1}{2} = 15$
$1 \times 15 = 15$

$$1x = 30 \times \frac{1}{2} = 15$$

$x = 15$ ml of Maalox

The fact that the bottle contained 8 oz of Maalox has nothing to do with the relationship between ml and 1 oz.

7. Give less than 1 ml.

Have   **Want to know**

gr $^1/_4$: 1 ml :: gr $^1/_6$: x ml   PROOF: $^1/_4 \times ^2/_3 = ^1/_6$

$$\frac{1}{4x} = \frac{1}{6}$$
                                        $1 \times ^1/_6 = ^1/_6$

$$\frac{1}{6} \div \frac{1}{4} = \frac{1}{6} \times \frac{4}{1} = {}^2/_3$$

$x = {}^2/_3$ ml

Answer must be a decimal. Therefore: $^2/_3 = 3\overline{)2.00}$

$$\begin{array}{r} .66 \\ 3\overline{)2.00} \\ \underline{1\ 8} \\ 20 \\ \underline{18} \\ 2 \end{array}$$

Give 0.66 ml of codeine sulfate SC.

4D Answer sheet

1. This is a two-step problem. First find out how many ml you are to give. Then figure how many minims per ml.

Have   **Want to know**

gr $^1/_{10}$: 1 ml :: gr $^1/_8$: x ml   PROOF: $1^1/_4 \times ^1/_{10} = ^1/_8$

$$\frac{{}^1\!/_{10}x}{{}^1\!/_{10}} = \frac{{}^1\!/_8}{{}^1\!/_{10}} = \frac{1}{8} \div \frac{1}{10} = \frac{1}{8} \times \frac{10}{1} = {}^5/_4 = 1^1/_4$$
                                  $1 \times ^1/_8 = ^1/_8$

$x = 1^1/_4$ ml

Since your problem is not completed, you may leave answer in fraction form or change it to a decimal.

You must memorize that there are 15 to 16 minims in 1 ml.

Have   **Want to know**

16 ♏ : 1 ml :: x ♏ : $1^1/_4$ ml   PROOF: $16 \times 1^1/_4 = 20$

$$1x = \frac{16}{1} \times \frac{5}{4} = \frac{80}{4} = 20$$
                                  $1 \times 20 = 20$

$x = 20$ minims

2. **Know**   **Want to know**

$8\ ʒ\ (dr):1\ ℥\ (oz)::x\ ʒ:{}^{1}/_{4}\ ℥$

PROOF: $8 \times {}^{1}/_{4} = 2$

$1 \times 2 = 2$

$1x = \dfrac{8}{1} \times \dfrac{1}{4} = \dfrac{8}{4} = 2$

$x = 2$ drams

3. This is a two-step problem.

   Have   **Want to know**

gr ${}^{1}/_{150}:{}^{1}/_{2}$ ml::gr ${}^{1}/_{200}:x$ ml

PROOF: ${}^{1}/_{2} \times {}^{1}/_{200} = {}^{1}/_{400}$

${}^{1}/_{150} \times {}^{3}/_{8} = {}^{1}/_{400}$

${}^{1}/_{150}x = \dfrac{1}{2} \times \dfrac{1}{200} = {}^{1}/_{400}$

$\dfrac{{}^{1}\!/\!\hspace{-2pt}\overline{150}x}{{}^{1}\!/\!\hspace{-2pt}\overline{150}} = \dfrac{{}^{1}/_{400}}{{}^{1}/_{150}} = \dfrac{1}{400} \times \dfrac{150}{1} = {}^{3}/_{8}$

$x = 0.37$ ml

You may either change fraction to decimal or leave it as it is for working out the remainder of the problem.

   Know   **Want to know**

16 ♏ :1 ml::x ♏ :${}^{3}/_{8}$ ml

PROOF: $1 \times 6 = 6$

$16 \times {}^{3}/_{8} = 6$

$1x = \dfrac{16}{1} \times \dfrac{3}{8} = \dfrac{48}{8} = 6$

$x = 6$ minims

4. **Have**   **Want to know**

gr $5:1$ tab.::gr $15:x$ tab.

PROOF: $5 \times 3 = 15$

$1 \times 15 = 15$

$5x = 15$

$x = 3$ tablets

5. **Know**   **Want to know**

$℥\ \text{i}:8\ ʒ::℥\ \overline{\text{ss}}:x\ ʒ$

PROOF: $1 \times 4 = 4$

$8 \times {}^{1}/_{2} = 4$

$x = 8 \times \dfrac{1}{2} = \dfrac{8}{2} = 4$

$x = 4$ drams

   Know   **Want to know**

$ʒ\ \text{i}:5$ ml::$ʒ$ ív:x ml

PROOF: $1 \times 20 = 20$

$5 \times 4 = 20$

$x = 5 \times 4 = 20$

$x = 20$ ml

Section 4 APOTHECARY SYSTEM QUIZ

1. Doctor has ordered Pantopon gr $^1/_6$ IM q.4h. p.r.n. The vial on hand is labeled Pantopon gr $^1/_3$ in 1 ml. How much will you give?

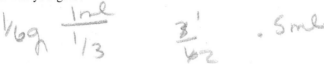

2. You are to give atropine gr $^1/_{200}$ as a preoperative medication. The vial on hand is labeled gr $^1/_{150}$ in 1 ml solution. How many ml will you give?

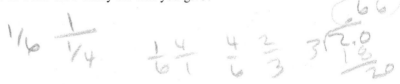

3. You are to give morphine sulfate (M.S.) gr $^1/_6$ with the above atropine. The morphine available is labeled gr $^1/_4$ in 1 ml. How many ml will you give?

4. Doctor has ordered ETH with codeine ℥ iii. This is equal to how many ml?

15 ml

5. You are to give codeine gr $^1/_8$. The drug available is labeled codeine gr $^1/_4$ per ml. How many ml will you give?

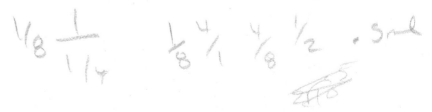

6. You are to give atropine gr $^1/_{200}$. On hand is a Tubex cartridge with gr $^1/_{150}$ in 0.5 ml. How many ml will you give? How many minims is this?

7. You have a vial of caffeine containing gr $1^1/_2$ per ml. You are to give gr $^3/_4$. How many ml will you give?

8. You are to give Gantrisin gr XV. On hand are Gantrisin tablets gr V. How many tablets will you give?

Section 4 Apothecary system quiz answer sheet _____

1. 0.5 ml
2. 0.75 ml
3. 0.66 ml
4. 15 ml
5. 0.5 ml
6. 0.37 ml and 6 ℳ
7. 0.5 ml
8. 3 tablets

Apothecary-metric conversions

UNIT A

Math objectives

1. *Memorize milligram/grain/gram equivalencies.*
2. *Memorize milliliter/quart/liter/pint and dram/minim/ounce equivalencies.*
3. *Round minims and drops to nearest correct number.*

Equivalency tables

VOLUME	WEIGHT
1000 milliliters (ml) = 1 liter (L) = 1 quart (qt) 1 ml = 1 cubic centimeter (cc) 500 ml = 1 pint (pt) 4 ml = 1 dram (dr or ʒ) or × 1 tsp = 4 or 5 ml 1 ml = 15 or 16 minims (♏) 1 ♏ = 1 drop (gtt) 30 ml = 1 ounce (ʒ)	*60 to 67 milligrams (mg) = grain (gr) 1 1 mg = gr *$^1/_{60}$ to $^1/_{67}$ 1 gram (g) = gr XV (15)

*The value 60 mg is more commonly used (see diagram below). The value gr $^1/_{60}$ = 1 mg is more commonly used than gr $^1/_{67}$.

A GOOD WAY TO REMEMBER:

"The Metric Clock"

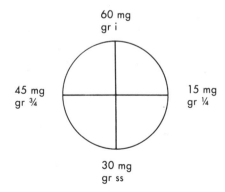

Section 5 answer sheets begin on p. 95.

RULE 1: When working with decimals, always remember to add a zero if there is no number before the decimal. This clarifies the decimal position and prevents medication errors.

EXAMPLE: 0.1 g is different from 1.0 g.

RULE 2: Apothecary is made definitive by adding a dot for clarification of the number one.

EXAMPLE: gr i (1) or gr viiss̄ (7½)

RULE 3: When working with the metric system, note that the symbol *follows* the Arabic number.

EXAMPLE: 0.5 g

When working with the apothecary system, note that roman numerals are frequently used. The symbol *precedes* the number.

EXAMPLE: gr xv

When proving answers from apothecary to metric, you will notice a slight difference (one tenth) because the apothecary system is not so accurate as the metric system. Proving answers *must* be done with the original answer and then rounded off if necessary.

EXAMPLE:

Know	Want to know	
1.0 g:gr 15::x g:gr 5		PROOF: $1.0 \times 5 = 5$
$15x = 5$		$15 \times 0.33 = 4.95 = 5$
$x = 0.333$ g		

Rounding off

RULE 4: Minims and drops are so small that it is impossible to divide them into parts. Therefore any remainder of 0.5 or above is given the next highest number.

EXAMPLE:

Minims   11.6   Give 12 ♏.
Drops   6.7 gtt   Give 7 gtt.

Syringes are calibrated in minims and tenths as well as ml. Therefore if the answer is 1.7 ml, do NOT round off to 2 ml. Tenths and hundredths can be measured accurately on syringes.

EXAMPLE: 1.68 ml   Give 1.7 ml in a 2 or 3 ml syringe.

The 8 in 1.68 is greater than 5, so the next highest number can be added to the 6, making the correct dosage 1.7 ml.

EXAMPLE: 0.73 ml   Give 0.73 ml.

Use a TB syringe for amounts less than 1 ml when a very precise dosage is indicated.

UNIT B

Math objective

Convert grains/grams/milligrams by using one-step ratio and proportion method.

5B Worksheet

MEMORIZE: 1 g = gr 15
60 mg = gr i

One-step problems

Use ratio and proportion, prove answers, and label answers:

1. gr 10 = _____ g

2. 0.5 g = gr _____

3. gr xxx = _____ g

4. 0.1 g = gr _____

5. gr viiss = _____ g

6. 3.0 g = gr _____

7. gr ³/₄ = _____ mg

8. 60 mg = gr _____

9. gr ¹/₄ = _____ mg

10. gr ¹/₃ = _____ mg

11. gr ¹/₁₅₀ = _____ mg

UNIT C

Math objective

Calculate metric-apothecary conversion problems.

5C Worksheet

Figure these in your head. Complete the following equivalents:

1. 1 mg = _____ g

2. 5 g = _____ mg

3. 1 g = gr _____

4. gr $7\frac{1}{2}$ = _____ g

5. 15 mg = gr _____

6. 1 L = _____ ml

7. 30 ml = _____ ʒ

8. 1 ml = _____ gtt

9. 2 ʒ = _____ ml

10. 1 cc = _____ ml

11. 1 kg = _____ g

12. gr i = _____ mg

13. gr iii = _____ mg

14. ʒ i = _____ ml

15. 1 tsp. = _____ ml

16. 1 gtt = _____ ♍

17. Which is smaller: mg or gr? _____

UNIT D _____

Math objective

Calculate metric-apothecary conversion problems.

5D Worksheet _____

MUST KNOW:

1 g = gr 15
gr i = 60 mg
℈ i = 30 ml
1 ml = 15 to 16 ♏

1. You are to give M.O.M. ℈ i̅s̅s̅. How many ml will you give?

   1.5 oz   *45 ml*

2. Doctor ordered atropine sulfate gr $^1/_{300}$ to be given on call to "O.R." On hand you have 0.50 mg per 0.5 ml. How many ml will you give?

   $\frac{1}{300} \times \frac{60mg}{1g} \times \frac{.5}{.50}$

3. You are ordered to give Demerol (meperidine hydrochloride) 0.025 g preoperatively @ 6:30 AM. Stock available is Demerol 50 mg/ml. How many ml will you give?

   $.025g \times \frac{60}{1g} \times \frac{ml}{50}$

4. Doctor ordered Demerol gr $^3/_4$. On hand you have a vial of Demerol labeled "75 mg/cc." How many ml will you give?

5. You are to give ASA (acetylsalicylic acid) 0.6 g. The tablets on hand are labeled "ASA gr v." How many tablets will you give?

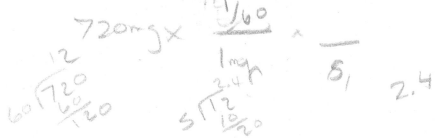

6. Doctor ordered 720 mg ASA for a temperature above 101° F. Your patient developed a fever of 101° F. How many tablets of ASA gr 5 per tablet will you give?

7. You are to give caffeine sodium benzoate gr viiss. You have an ampule labeled "caffeine sodium benzoate 0.5 g in 2.0 cc." How many ml will you give?

8. You have a 2 ml ampule of caffeine Na benzoate containing gr viiss. If the physician orders gr V, you will give how many minims?

UNIT E

Math objective

Calculate metric-apothecary conversion problems.

5E Worksheet

1. The physician ordered gr $^1/_{200}$ scopolamine SC injection. On hand is a vial of scopolamine that reads "1 ml = gr $^1/_{150}$." How many ml would you give?

$$\frac{1}{200} \times \frac{1}{\frac{1}{150}} \qquad .75$$

2. In the narcotic box the morphine is labeled "M.S. gr $^1/_4$ per 1 cc." The physician ordered M.S. gr $^1/_6$. How many ml would you give (to nearest tenth)?
   Before you begin this problem, can you tell if you will give more or less than 1 ml?

$$\frac{1}{6} \times \frac{1}{\frac{1}{4}} \qquad \frac{4}{6} \qquad \frac{2}{3}$$

3. The physician ordered codeine gr $^1/_2$ oral. On hand are tablets 15 mg. How many tablets would you give?

$$.5 \times \frac{60}{1 \text{ gr}} \qquad \frac{60}{.5}{300} \qquad 2$$

4. Penicillin 300,000 U IM is ordered every 4 hours. On hand is a 10 ml vial of penicillin labeled "400,000 U per 1 ml." How many minims would you give for 1 dose?

$$300,000 \times \frac{1}{400,000} \qquad 3 \times \frac{1}{4}$$

$$400 \overline{)10} \qquad 400 \overline{)300,000}$$

91

5. Gantrisin 0.50 g (oral) is ordered. On hand is Gantrisin 250 mg per tablet. How many tablets would you give?

$$.50g \times \frac{1000 mg}{1g} \times \frac{}{250} = 2 \, tabs$$

6. Demerol 75 mg IM is ordered stat. On hand is Demerol 100 mg per 2 ml. How many ml would you give (nearest tenth)?

$$75mg \times \frac{2}{100mg} \qquad 1.5 \, ml$$

7. Atropine gr $^1/_{300}$ by injection is ordered for a patient going to surgery. The nurse has a bottle from stock labeled "scopolamine gr $^1/_{150}$." How many minims of scopolamine would you give?

$1cc = 15 min$

$$^1/_{300} \, gr \times \frac{}{^1/_{150}} \qquad \begin{array}{c} .5 \\ 7-8 \, minims \end{array}$$

8. Chloral hydrate gr viiss is ordered for sleep. On hand is a bottle marked "chloral hydrate." One tablet is 0.25 g. How many tablets would you give?

37.5

$$7.5 \, gr \times \frac{1 gm}{15 gr} \times \frac{}{.25} \qquad .2 \qquad 2$$

$$.5$$

UNIT F

Math objective

Calculate metric-apothecary conversion problems.

5F Worksheet

Prove and label answers:

1. Atropine gr $^{1}/_{150}$ per ml is found in stock. The physician ordered gr $^{1}/_{200}$ to be given by injection. How many minims would you give?

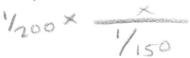

2. Maalox is ordered ℥ s̄s̄ q.2h. How many ml would you give? How many ml will you give in 24 hours?

3. Ordered was "tincture of belladonna minims IX in $^{1}/_{2}$ glass water." How many drops would you use?

9 minims

4. How many ml of water would you use for the above if the glass holds 6 oz?

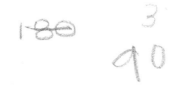

5. Elixir of phenobarbital 8 ml was ordered. How many teaspoons is this? How many ℥ is this?

8 ml

1 ½ tesp   1.5 drams.

6. The physician ordered Kantrex 0.2 g q.4hr. by injection. The vial of Kantrex is labeled "Add 5 ml sterile water for 1 g per 2 ml." How many ml would you give?

.2g × $\frac{2}{1g}$ .4 ml

7. Ordered was 0.05 g Talwin P.O. On hand was Talwin 100 mg tablets. How many tablets will you give?

.05g × $\frac{1000}{1g}$ × $\frac{}{100}$ ½ tab

Section 5 APOTHECARY-METRIC CONVERSIONS ANSWER SHEETS

5B Answer sheet

1. **Know**   **Want to know**

    1.0 g:gr 15::x g:gr 10

    $15x = 10 = 10 \div 15 = 0.66$

    $x = 0.66$ g

    PROOF: $15 \times 0.66 = 9.9 = 10$

             $1 \times 10 = 10$

2. **Know**   **Want to know**

    1.0 g:gr 15::0.5 g:gr x

    $1x = 15 \times 0.5 = 7.5$

    $x = 7.5$

    PROOF: $15 \times 0.5 = 7.5$

             $1 \times 7.5 = 7.5$

3. **Know**   **Want to know**

    1.0 g:gr 15::x g:gr 30

    $15x = 30$

    $x = 2$ g

    PROOF: $15 \times 2 = 30$

             $1 \times 30 = 30$

4. **Know**   **Want to know**

    1.0 g:gr 15::0.1 g:gr x

    $1x = 1.5$

    $x = $ gr 1.5

    PROOF: $15 \times 0.1 = 1.5$

             $1 \times 1.5 = 1.5$

5. **Know**   **Want to know**

    1.0 g:gr 15::x g:gr 7$\frac{1}{2}$

    $15x = 7\frac{1}{2}$

    $x = 0.5$ g

    PROOF: $15 \times 0.5 = 7.5$

             $1 \times 7.5 = 7.5$

6. **Know**   **Want to know**

    1.0 g:gr 15::3.0 g:gr x

    $1.0x = 45.0$

    $x = $ gr 45.0

    PROOF: $15 \times 3.0 = 45$

             $1.0 \times 45.0 = 45$

7. **Know**   **Want to know**

60.0 mg : gr i : : x mg : gr $^3/_4$

$1x = 60 \times {}^3/_4 = 45$

$x = 45$ mg

PROOF: $1 \times 45 = 45$

$60 \times {}^3/_4 = 45$

8. **Know**   **Want to know**

60 mg : gr i : : 60 mg : gr x

$60x = 60$

$x = $ gr 1

PROOF: $1 \times 60 = 60$

$60 \times 1 = 60$

9. **Know**   **Want to know**

60 mg : gr 1 : : x mg : gr $^1/_4$

$1x = 60 \times {}^1/_4 = 15$

$x = 15$ mg

PROOF: $1 \times 15 = 15$

$60 \times {}^1/_4 = 15$

10. **Know**   **Want to know**

60 mg : gr 1 : : x mg : gr $^1/_3$

$1x = 60 \times {}^1/_3 = 20$

$x = 20$ mg

PROOF: $1 \times 20 = 20$

$60 \times {}^1/_3 = 20$

11. **Know**   **Want to know**

60 mg : gr 1 : : x mg : gr $^1/_{150}$

$1x = 60 \times \dfrac{1}{150} = {}^2/_5 = 5\overline{)2.0} \; \dfrac{0.4}{}$

$\underline{2\ 0}$

$x = 0.4$ mg

PROOF: $1 \times 0.4 = 0.4$

$60 \times {}^1/_{150} = {}^2/_5 = 0.4$

5C Answer sheet

Use conversion tables for proof.

1. 0.001 g
2. 5000 mg
3. gr 15
4. 0.5 g
5. gr $^1/_4$
6. 1000 ml

7. 1 oz
8. 15 to 16 gtt
9. 8 ml
10. 1 ml
11. 1000 g
12. 60 mg

13. 180 mg
14. 30 ml
15. 5 ml
16. 1 ℔
17. Milligrams are smaller than grains (gr i = 60 mg).

5D Answer sheet

REMEMBER: *Know* or *have* always goes on the *left*.

1. ℥ i : 30 ml :: ℥ 1½ : x ml

   $$1x = 30 \times 1\frac{1}{2} = \frac{15}{1} \times \frac{3}{4} = 45$$

   $x = 45$ ml

   PROOF: $30 \times 1\frac{1}{2} = 45$
   $1 \times 45 = 45$

2. This is a two-step problem. Must change gr $^1/_{300}$ to mg because that is what you have on hand.

Know	Want to know

   60 mg : gr i :: x mg : gr $^1/_{300}$

   PROOF: $1 \times ^1/_5 = ^1/_5$
   $60 \times ^1/_{300} = ^1/_5$

   $$1x = \frac{1}{300} \times \frac{60}{1} = ^1/_5$$

   $x = ^1/_5$ mg   Change $^1/_5$ to a decimal because mg is a metric measure and metric is a decimal system; so: $1 \div 5 = 0.2$ mg.

Have	Want to know

   0.5 mg : 0.5 ml :: 0.2 mg : x ml
   $0.50x = 0.10$
   $x = 0.2$ ml   Give 0.2 ml of atropine.

   PROOF: $0.50 \times 0.2 = 0.1$
   $0.5 \times 0.2 = 0.1$

3. | Know | Want to know |
   |---|---|

   1000 mg : 1 g :: x mg : 0.025 g
   $1x = 1000 \times 0.025$
   $x = 25$ mg

   PROOF: $1000 \times 0.025 = 25$
   $1 \times 25 = 25$

Have	Want to know

   50 mg : 1 ml :: 25 mg : x ml
   $50x = 25$
   $x = 0.5$ ml   Give 0.5 ml of Demerol.

   PROOF: $1 \times 25 = 25$
   $50 \times 0.5 = 25$

NOTE: Do *not* round off ml or cc to whole numbers. Syringes are marked to give tenths and hundredths. Check the calibrations on your syringes.

4. | Know | Want to know |
   |---|---|

   60 mg : gr i :: x mg : gr $^3/_4$
   $1x = 60 \times ^3/_4 = 45$
   $x = 45$ mg

   PROOF: $1 \times 45 = 45$
   $60 \times ^3/_4 = 45$

Have	Want to know

   75 mg : 1 ml :: 45 mg : x ml
   $75x = 45$
   $x = 0.6$ ml

   PROOF: $1 \times 45 = 45$
   $75 \times 0.6 = 45$

5. **Know**   **Want to know**

1 g:gr $15::0.6$ g:gr x PROOF: $15 \times 0.6 = 9$

$1x = 9$ $1 \times 9 = 9$

$x = $ gr 9

Have   **Want to know**

gr $5:1$ tab. $::$ gr $9:x$ tab.   PROOF: $1 \times 9 = 9$

$5x = 9$ $5 \times 1.8 = 9$

$x = 1.8$ tablets   Give 2 tablets of gr v each tablet.

Can you give $^8/_{10}$ of a tablet? Not very easily, so the only thing to do is to give 2 tablets of gr v.

6. **Know**   **Want to know**

60 mg:gr i$::720$ mg:gr x PROOF: $720 \times 1 = 720$

$60x = 720$ $60 \times 12 = 720$

$x = 12$ gr

Have   **Want to know**

gr $5:1$ tab. $::$ gr $12:x$ tab.   PROOF: $1 \times 12 = 12$

$5x = 12$ $5 \times 2.4 = 12$

$x = 2.4$ tablets   Give $2\frac{1}{2}$ tablets of gr 5 each.

7. **Know**   **Want to know**

1 g:gr $15::x$ g:gr $7\frac{1}{2}$ PROOF: $15 \times 0.5 = 7.5$

$15x = 7\frac{1}{2}$ $7.5 \times 1 = 7.5$

$x = 0.5$ g

Have   **Want to know**

0.5 g:2.0 cc$::0.5$ g:x cc   PROOF: $2 \times 0.5 = 1$

$0.5x = 1.0$ $0.5 \times 2 = 1$

$x = 2$ cc (ml)

8. **Have**   **Want to know**

gr $7\frac{1}{2}:2$ ml$::$gr $5:x$ ml   PROOF: $2 \times 5 = 10$

$7\frac{1}{2}x = 2 \times 5 = 10$ $7\frac{1}{2} \times 1\frac{1}{3} = 10$

$x = 1\frac{1}{3}$ ml   Now change this to minims.

Know   **Want to know**

15 ♏ :1 ml$::x$ ♏ :$1\frac{1}{3}$ ml   PROOF: $1 \times 20 = 20$

$1x = 15 \times 1\frac{1}{3} = 15 \times \frac{4}{3} = 20$ $15 \times 1\frac{1}{3} = 20$

$x = 20$ minims

5E Answer sheet

1. **Have**   **Want to know**

   gr $^1/_{150}$:1 ml::gr $^1/_{200}$:x ml   PROOF: $^1/_{150} \times {}^3/_4 = {}^1/_{200}$

    $1 \times {}^1/_{200} = {}^1/_{200}$

   $^1/_{150}x = {}^1/_{200} = \dfrac{1}{200} \div \dfrac{1}{150} = \dfrac{1}{200} \times \dfrac{150}{1} = {}^3/_4$ ml

   $x = {}^3/_4$ ml

   Change $^3/_4$ ml to metric (decimal) 0.75

2. **Have**   **Want to know**

   gr $^1/_4$:1 ml::gr $^1/_6$:x ml   PROOF: $1 \times {}^1/_6 = {}^1/_6$

   $^1/_4x = {}^1/_6$ $^1/_4 \times {}^2/_3 = {}^1/_6$

   $x = {}^2/_3$ ml or $0.66 = 0.7$ ml

   Change fraction to metric (decimal).

3. **Know**   **Want to know**

   60 mg:gr i::x mg:gr $^1/_2$ PROOF: $1 \times 30 = 30$

   $1x = 60 \times {}^1/_2 = 30$ $60 \times {}^1/_2 = 30$

   $x = 30$ mg

   Have   **Want to know**

   15 mg:1 tab.::30 mg:x tab.   PROOF: $1 \times 30 = 30$

   $15x = 30$ $15 \times 2 = 30$

   $x = 2$ tablets

4. **Have**   **Want to know**

   400,000 U:1 ml::300,000 U:x ml   PROOF: $1 \times 300{,}000 = 300{,}000$

    $400{,}000 \times 0.75 = 300{,}000$

   $\dfrac{\cancel{400{,}000}x}{\cancel{400{,}000}} = \dfrac{\cancel{300{,}000}}{\cancel{400{,}000}} = \dfrac{3}{4} = 3 \div 4 = 0.75$

   $x = 0.75$ ml

   Know   **Want to know**

   15 ♏:1 ml::x ♏:0.75 ml   PROOF: $1 \times 11 = 11$

   $1x = 15 \times 0.75 = 11.25$ $15 \times 0.75 = 11.25$

   $x = 11$ minims

5. **Know**   **Want to know**

    1000 mg : 1 g :: x mg : 0.50 g   PROOF: $1 \times 500 = 500$

    $1x = 500$ mg $1000 \times 0.50 = 500$

    $x = 500$ mg

    Have   **Want to know**

    250 mg : 1 tab. :: 500 mg : x tab.   PROOF: $1 \times 500 = 500$

    $250x = 500$ $250 \times 2 = 500$

    $x = 2$ tablets

6. **Have**   **Want to know**

    100 mg : 2 ml :: 75 mg : x ml   PROOF: $2 \times 75 = 150$

    $100x = 150$ $100 \times 1.5 = 150$

    $x = 1.5$ ml

7. None. We hope you won't give scopolamine when atropine was ordered.

8. **Know**   **Want to know**

    1 g : gr 15 :: x g : gr $7\frac{1}{2}$ PROOF: $15 \times 0.5 = 7.5$

    $15x = 7\frac{1}{2}$ $1 \times 7\frac{1}{2} = 7\frac{1}{2}$

    $1x = \dfrac{7\frac{1}{2}}{15} = \frac{1}{2}$

    $x = 0.5$ g

    Have   **Want to know**

    0.25 g : 1 tab. :: 0.5 g : x tab.   PROOF: $1 \times 0.5 = 0.5$

    $0.25x = 0.5$ $0.25 \times 2 = 0.5$

    $1x = \dfrac{0.5}{0.25} = 2$

    $x = 2$ tablets

1. **Have**   **Want to know**

   gr $^1/_{150}$:1 ml::gr $^1/_{200}$:x ml   PROOF: $1 \times ^1/_{200} = ^1/_{200}$

   $^1/_{150}x = ^1/_{200} \div ^1/_{150} = ^1/_{200} \times ^{150}/_1 = ^3/_4$ $^1/_{150} \times ^3/_4 = ^1/_{200}$

   $x = ^3/_4 = 0.75$ ml   Give 0.75 ml of atropine.

   Know   **Want to know**

   16 ♏ :1 ml::x ♏ :$^3/_4$ ml   PROOF: $1 \times 12 = 12$

   $1x = 16 \times ^3/_4 = 12$ $16 \times ^3/_4 = 12$

   $x = 12$ ♏

2. **Know**   **Want to know**

   ℥ i:30 ml::℥ $^1/_2$:x ml   PROOF: $30 \times ^1/_2 = 15$

   $1x = 30 \times ^1/_2 = 15$ $1 \times 15 = 15$

   $x = 15$ ml

   Know   **Want to know**

   15 ml:2 hr::x ml:24 hr   PROOF: $2 \times 180 = 360$

   $2x = 360$ $15 \times 24 = 360$

   $x = 180$ ml in 24 hr

3. **Know**   **Want to know**

   1 ♏ :1 gtt::9 ♏ :x gtt   PROOF: $9 \times 1 = 9$

   $1x = 9$ $1 \times 9 = 9$

   $x = 9$ gtt

4. **Know**   **Want to know**

   30 ml:1 oz::x ml:6 oz   PROOF: $1 \times 180 = 180$

   $1x = 180$ $6 \times 30 = 180$

   $x = 180$ ml

   Have   **Want to know**

   180 ml:6 oz::x ml:3 oz ($^1/_2$ glass)   PROOF: $6 \times 90 = 540$

   $6x = 540$ $3 \times 180 = 540$

   $x = 90$ ml

5. **Know**   **Want to know**

    4 ml : 1 tsp. : : 8 ml : x tsp.

    $4x = 8$

    $x = 2$ tsp.

    PROOF: $1 \times 8 = 8$

              $4 \times 2 = 8$

    Know   **Want to know**

    1 dr : 4 ml : : x dr : 8 ml

    $4x = 8$

    $x = 2$ drams

    PROOF: $1 \times 8 = 8$

              $4 \times 2 = 8$

6. **Have**   **Want to know**

    1 g : 2 ml : : 0.2 g : x ml

    $x = 2 \times 0.2 = 0.4$

    $x = 0.4$ ml

    PROOF: $1 \times 0.4 = 0.4$

              $2 \times 0.2 = 0.4$

7. **Know**   **Want to know**

    1000 mg : 1 g : : x mg : 0.05 g

    $1x = 1000 \times 0.05 = 50$

    $x = 50$ mg

    PROOF: $1 \times 50 = 50$

              $1000 \times 0.05 = 50$

    Know   **Want to know**

    100 mg : 1 tab. : : 50 mg : x tab.

    $100x = 50 \div 100 = \frac{1}{2}$

    $x = 0.5$ tablet or $\frac{1}{2}$ tablet

    PROOF: $50 \times 1 = 50$

              $100 \times \frac{1}{2} = 50$

Section 5 APOTHECARY-METRIC QUIZ

Use ratio and proportion, prove, and label:

1. gr 10 = _____.67_____ g

   15gr = 1gm

5. gr 5 = _____.34_____ g

   5grx $\frac{1}{15g}$

   10gr× $\frac{1}{15g}$

2. 0.5 g = gr _____15_____

   .5gm × $\frac{15gr}{1gm}$

6. gr viiss = _____.5_____ g

   7.5gr× $\frac{1}{15gr}$

3. gr xxx = _____2_____ g

   30gr × $\frac{1}{15}$

7. 3 g = gr _____45_____

   3gm× $\frac{15g}{1gm}$

4. 90 mg = gr _____1.5_____

   9mg× $\frac{1/60}{1mg}$ 1½

8. Ordered: tincture of belladonna minims ix in ½ glass water. How many drops will you give?

   9 gtts

9. Ordered: M.S. gr ⅙. On hand: M.S. gr ¼ ml. Give _____ ml.

   ⅙ × $\frac{1}{14}$ $\frac{4}{6}$ ⅔

   .7ml

10. Ordered: atropine gr ¹/₃₀₀. On hand: atropine gr ¹/₁₅₀ per 0.5 ml. Give _____ ml.

   ¹/₃₀₀ × $\frac{.5}{1/150}$ .25

   $\frac{150}{300}$

103

Section 5 Apothecary-metric quiz answer sheet _____

1. 0.67 g
2. gr 7½
3. 2 g
4. gr 1½

5. 0.33 g
6. 0.5 g
7. gr 45

8. 9 gtt
9. 0.66 ml
10. 0.25 ml

Intravenous calculations: drop factors and basic titrations

Math objectives

1. *Memorize two-step formula for calculating IV flow rates.*
2. *Given doctor's order for IV solution, calculate milligrams per hour.*
3. *Using drop factor, calculate drops per minute.*
4. *Memorize drop factor for microdrip tubing.*
5. *Determine whether to start at step 1 or step 2 of IV rate calculation.*
6. *Calculate simple IV titration problems.*

UNIT A

IV flow rate

There are two steps in IV calculations. The first step is to find out how many ml per hour the IV infusion requires. The second step is to calculate how many drops per minute are needed to give the patient the ml/hr you know he or she should have.

Analyze your problem. If the doctor ordered the IV to infuse for 8 hours, you must begin at step 1 to figure out how many ml/hr the patient must have. If the doctor writes the order and *tells you* the IV is to run at 75 ml/hr, then you can start at step 2.

Step 1: How to calculate milliliters per hour

Doctor ordered 2000 ml D5W (dextrose 5% in water) to be infused in 8 hours. The problem is to find out how many ml/hr the patient must receive for the 2000 ml to be absorbed or infused in 8 hours.

FORMULA:

$$\frac{\text{Total volume (TV)}}{\text{Total time (TT)}} = \text{ml/hr}$$

$$\frac{\text{Total volume}}{\text{Total time}} = \frac{2000 \text{ ml}}{8 \text{ hr}} = \text{ml/hr}$$

$$\frac{\text{TV}}{\text{TT}} = \frac{2000}{8} = 2000 \div 8 = 250 \text{ ml/hr}$$

Section 6 answer sheets begin on p. 121.

We now know that to get 2000 ml of fluid in 8 hours the patient must get 250 ml/hr. Now you must calculate how many drops you need per *minute* so the patient will receive 250 ml/hr.

Drop factor

The drop factor is the number of drops in 1 ml (or 1 cc). The diameter of the tube where the drop enters the drip chamber varies from one manufacturer to another. The bigger the tube, the fatter the drop; thus it may take only 10 gtt to make up a ml. The smallest unit is the microdrop (60 gtt/ml). This is used for people who can tolerate only small amounts of fluid. Drop factors of 10, 12, 13, 15, 20, and 60 (microdrip) are the most common. The drop factor is found on the IV tubing box.

Step 2: How to calculate drops per minute

FORMULA:

$$\frac{\text{Drop factor or gtt/ml (from IV box)}}{\text{Time in minutes}} \times \text{Total hourly volume (V/hr)} = \text{gtt/min}$$

If the drop factor is 10 and you want the IV to infuse at 250 ml/hr, how many drops per minute will you time on your watch?

$$\frac{\text{Drop factor (Df)}}{\text{Time (min)}} \times \text{V/hr or} \frac{10\ (\text{Df})}{60\ (\text{min})} \times 250\ \text{ml (V/hr)} = \text{gtt/min}$$

$$\frac{10}{60} \times \frac{250}{1} = \frac{1}{6} \times \frac{250}{1} = \frac{250}{6} = 41.6\ \text{or}\ 42\ \text{drops/min}$$

Summary: Two-step IV flow rate calculations

1. $\dfrac{\text{T V}}{\text{T T}} = \text{ml/hr}$

2. $\dfrac{\text{Df}}{\text{Min}} \times \text{V/hr} = \text{gtt/min}$ Remember to reduce fraction before multiplying.

   or

   $\dfrac{\text{D}}{\text{M}} \times \text{V} = \text{gtt/min}$ DMV (Department of Motor Vehicles) may be easier to remember.

REMEMBER: Reduce the fraction $\dfrac{\text{Df}}{\text{Min}}$ or $\dfrac{\text{D}}{\text{M}}$ *before* multiplying times the volume.

EXAMPLE:
Which would you rather calculate?

a. $\dfrac{12}{60} \times 60$ or   b. $\dfrac{1}{5} \times 60$

The reduced fraction is easier to calculate.

Abbreviations for common intravenous solutions

NS	Normal saline 0.9%
1/2 NS	Normal saline 0.45%
D/RL	Dextrose with Ringer's lactate solution
D5W or 5% D/W	Dextrose 5% in water
RL	Ringer's lactate solution (electrolytes)
Isolytes	Electrolyte solutions

UNIT B

Math objectives

1. *Calculate IV flow rates.*
2. *Determine whether to start with step 1 or step 2 of IV rate calculations.*

6B Worksheet*

1. Doctor ordered 1000 ml to be infused in 8 hr. How many gtt/min if the drop factor is 10?

   Start at step _____ .

   60×8 $\dfrac{1000}{480} \times 10 = 20.8$

2. Ordered: 200 ml is to be infused in an hour. If drop factor is 12, how many gtt/min?

   Start at step _____ .

   $\dfrac{200 \, ml}{60} \times 12 = 399$

3. Doctor ordered 100 ml to be infused in 30 min. How many gtt/min if drop factor is 10?

   Start at step _____ .

   $\dfrac{100}{30} \times 10 = 33.3$

4. Order calls for 1500 ml to be infused in 12 hr. If drop factor is 15, how many gtt/min?

   Start at step _____ .

   $\dfrac{1500}{720} \times 15 = 31$

5. Doctor ordered 50 ml to be infused in an hour. How many gtt/min with microdrip?

   $\dfrac{50}{60} \times 60 \qquad 50 \, gtts$

---

*FORMULA: $\dfrac{TV}{TT} = $ ml/hr

$\dfrac{D}{M} \times V = $ gtt/min

108

6. Doctor ordered 1500 ml to be infused in 8 hr. How many ml/hr?

187.5

a. How many gtt/min with drop factor of 10?

$$\frac{1500}{480} \times 10 \qquad 31.25$$

b. How many gtt/min with drop factor of 13?

$$\frac{1500}{480} \times 13 = 40.6$$

7. Doctor ordered 75 ml to be infused in 45 min. Drop factor is 10. How many gtt/min?

$$\frac{75}{45} \times 10 = 16.6$$

UNIT C

Math objective

Calculate IV flow rates.

6C Worksheet

1. You have 2000 ml 5% D/W being infused for 24 hr. Drop factor is 10. How many ml/hr?

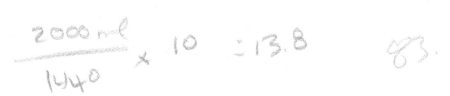

$$\frac{2000\ ml}{1440} \times 10 = 13.8 \qquad 83.$$

2. You have 1500 ml NS. Drop factor is 15. Solution is to be given for an 8 hr period. How many ml/hr? How many gtt/min?

3. Solution of 3000 ml D5W is being infused for 24 hr with 1.5 g carbenicillin. Drop factor is 60 (microdrip). How many gtt/min? On which step will you begin?

4. You have 500 ml 0.45% NS infusing for 4 hr. Drop factor is 13. How many gtt/min?

5. Doctor ordered 1000 ml to be infused for 12 hr on microdrip. How many gtt/min will you regulate the flow?

6. Order calls for 100 ml gentamycin to be infused within 30 min. Drop factor is 12. How many gtt/min?

7. Doctor ordered 2000 ml for 24 hr. Drop factor is 15. How many gtt/min?

8. Ordered: 150 ml D5W is to be infused for 10 hr on a microdrip. How many gtt/min?

9. Doctor ordered 1500 ml of Ringer's lactate solution to run for 12 hr. How many ml/hr? Drop factor is 15. How many gtt/min?

10. Write your two-step formula again.

Step 1

Step 2

UNIT D _____

Math objective

Calculate IV flow rates.

6D Worksheet _____

1. Doctor ordered 100 ml/hr. How many gtt/min if drop factor is 10? (Start at step 1 or step 2?)

2. Ordered: 1000 ml to be infused in 6 hr. How many gtt/min if drop factor is 15? (Start at step 1 or step 2?)

3. Doctor ordered 50 ml to be infused in 30 min. How many gtt/min if drop factor is 10? (Start at step 1 or 2?)

4. Order calls for 100 ml to be infused in 60 min. How many gtt/min if a microdrip is used? (Start at step 1 or step 2?)

5. Doctor ordered 2000 ml to be infused in 12 hr. Drop factor is 60.

   a. How many ml/hr?

   b. How many gtt/min?

6. Ordered: 100 ml to be infused in 30 min. Drop factor is 12. How many gtt/min?

7. Doctor ordered 1500 ml 0.45% NS in 24 hr. Drop factor is 10. How many gtt/min?

8. Order calls for 500 ml in 8 hr by microdrip. How many gtt/min?

UNIT E

Math objective

Calculate IV flow rates.

6E Worksheet

1. Doctor ordered Keflin 4 g in 100 ml IV piggyback to be infused over 1 hr. If drop factor is 10, how many gtt/min?

2. Order calls for ampicillin 500 mg in 50 ml IV piggyback to be infused in 20 min. How many gtt/min if drop factor is 15?

3. Doctor ordered gentamycin 80 mg in 50 ml IV piggyback to be infused in 30 min. How many gtt/min if drop factor is 60?

4. Order calls for Aq. penicillin 600,000 U. in 100 ml IV piggyback to be infused in 1 hr. If drop factor is 12, how many gtt/min?

UNIT F

Math objective

Solve titration problems by sequencing steps using deductive reasoning.

Hints for solving titration problems*

As you read the entire problem, number the steps in sequence. Begin by converting pounds (lb) to kilograms (kg); then proceed to convert milligrams (mg) to micrograms (μg)† [or opposite, depending upon problem] if necessary. Calculate the maximum μg/min (if applicable), and then determine how many minutes or hours the medication will take to infuse. The gtt/min the patient is to receive will be the final step. Variations of this sequence are used, depending upon the problem. Answers to the following problem are to be calculated using the microdrip (60 gtt/ml or 60 ml/hr). A calculator will be useful.

EXAMPLE:

Doctor ordered 200 mg Intropin (dopamine HCl) IV drip. Directions read: "8 μg/kg/min starting with 200 mg dissolved in 250 ml 5% D/W." On hand is a 5 ml vial containing 400 mg Intropin. The patient weighs 210 lb. Current IV is infusing at 100 ml/hr (microdrip).

How long will it take for the ordered medication to be infused? What is the gtt/min rate? Will you have to change the IV rate?

Steps to solve problem

1. Convert lb to kg. (Calculate to tenths.)
2. Convert μg (or mcg) to what the label reads (mg).
3. Calculate how many mg/min are needed for the kg of body weight.
4. Calculate how many hours or minutes it will take to infuse the ordered amount of medication.
5. Calculate how many ml of medication you will add to the recommended dilution of solvent and figure total amount (volume) to be infused.
6. Use the microdrip drop factor to calculate gtt/min.

---

*Refer to Children's Dosages, Section 11, Units A and B, for skill building.
†The abbreviations μg and mcg are used interchangeably.

ANSWERS:

Step 1: lb to kg

1 kg:2.2 lb::x kg:210 lbs   PROOF: $2.2 \times 95.4 = 209.8$

$2.2x = 210$ $1 \times 210 = 210$

$x = 95.4$ kg

Step 2: μg to mg

1 mg:1000 μg::x mg:8 μg   PROOF: $1000 \times 0.008 = 8$

$1000x = 8$ $1 \times 8 = 8$

$x = 0.008$ mg

Step 3: mg/kg/min

0.008 mg:1 kg::x mg:95.4 kg   PROOF: $1 \times 0.76 = 0.76$

$x = 0.008 \times 95.4 = 0.76$ $0.008 \times 95.4 = 0.76$

$x = 0.76$ mg/min for a 95.4 kg person

Step 4: min/ordered dose

0.76 mg:1 min::200 mg:x min   PROOF: $0.76 \times 263.15 = 199.9$

$0.76x = 200$ $1 \times 200 = 200$

$x = 263$ min $\div$ 60 = 4 hr and 24 min

Step 5: ml of medication

5 ml:400 mg::x ml:200 mg   PROOF: $400 \times 2.5 = 1000$

$400x = 5 \times 200 = 1000$ $5 \times 200 = 1000$

$400x = 1000$

$x = 2.5$ ml   Add x to 250 ml = 252.5 ml total.

Step 6: gtt/min

$$\frac{60}{263} \times 252.5 = \frac{15150}{263} = 57.6 = 58 \text{ gtt/min}$$

Current IV rate is 100 ml/hr = 100 gtt/min (microdrip).

Decrease IV rate to infuse 58 gtt/min.

UNIT G

Math objective

Titrate mg/kg, mg/min, μg/min, and calculate flow rate and administration time.

6G Worksheet

1. Doctor ordered dobutamine HCl (Dobutrex) 200 mg IV drip. Label reads "250 mg/20 ml." Further dilute to at least 50 ml and administer as a continuous infusion at the usual dose of 2.5 to 10 μg/kg/min. The patient weighed 155 lb today. The current IV is infusing at 125 ml/hr. What will be the correct flow rate (gtt/min) for this patient?

Steps to solve problem

   1. How much does the patient weigh in kg? Calculate to tenths. Do *not* round.
   2. At the above rates of administration, which will give the maximum rate per minute (μg/kg/min)?
   3. How many μg are in 200 mg?
   4. How many μg/min can the patient safely receive?
   5. How many minutes or hours will it take to deliver the total ordered dose?
   6. After adding the medication to the 50 ml, what will be the total volume infused?
   7. What will be the flow rate in gtt/min?
   8. Do you have to change the current IV rate?

2. Doctor ordered quinidine sulfate 250 mg IV drip for arrhythmia. Label reads "80 mg/ml in a 10 ml vial." Dilute the 10 ml vial (800 mg) to 50 ml, using 40 ml D5W as a diluent. Give at the rate of 1 ml (16 mg) per minute.
   How long will it take to administer 250 mg? The current IV is infusing at 75 ml/hr.

Steps to solve problem

   1. How many ml of solution will need to be infused to deliver 250 mg?
   2. How many minutes will it take to deliver the ordered amount of medication?
   3. How many gtt/min will be infused?
   4. Will you have to readjust the current rate?

Section 6, Unit G answer sheet begins on p. 126.

3. Doctor ordered sodium nitroprusside (Nipride) 50 mg IV drip stat. Label reads: "Usual dose is 3 μg/kg/min. Each 50 mg must be dissolved with 2 to 3 ml of D5W. Further dilute in a minimum of 250 ml of D5W for administration. Protect bottle and tubing from sunlight. A potent, rapid-acting antihypertensive." Current IV is infusing at 85 ml/hr. The patient weighs 165 lb.
How many gtt/min is safe for this patient?

Steps to solve problem

1. How much does patient weigh in kg? Calculate to tenths. Do *not* round.
2. How many μg are in 50 mg?
3. How many μg/kg/min can the patient safely receive?
4. After adding the medication to 250 ml D5W, what will be the total volume infused?
5. How many minutes or hours will it take to deliver the total ordered dose?
6. What will be the flow rate in gtt/min?
7. Do you have to change the current IV rate?

4. Doctor ordered lidocaine 4 mg/min IV drip for arrhythmia. Literature reads: "For a continuous infusion administer at the rate of 1 to 4 mg/min (20 to 50 μg/kg/min in the average 70 kg man). To prepare IV solution, add 1 or 2 g Xylocaine HCl to 1 liter of 5% D/W. 1 g in 1000 ml = 0.1% solution. 2 g in 1000 ml = 0.2% solution. Each ml will contain approximately 1 to 2 mg; therefore 1 to 4 ml/min will provide 1 to 4 mg lidocaine HCl. No more than 200 to 300 mg should be administered during a 1 hr period. Monitor patient on ECG." Patient weighs 182 lb. Current IV rate is 100 ml/hr. Use the 0.1% dilution.
   a. Is 4 mg/min a safe dose for a 1 hr period?
   b. How many ml/hr will deliver 4 mg/min?
   c. Will you have to change the IV rate?

Steps to solve problem

1. Convert lb to kg.
2. Calculate the safe maximum μg and mg/kg/min for patient. Is 4 mg/min a safe dose?
3. Using the 4 mg/min order, how many *mg* will be infused in 1 hour? Is this a safe dose for 1 hour?
4. Use 0.1% dilution to determine g, mg, and μg in 1 ml.
5. How many *ml*/hr will be infused? How many gtt/min (microdrip)?

UNIT H

Math objective

Calculate units per minute for insulin and heparin IV infusions.

Medications can be infused by IV bolus (direct IV) or by piggyback/volutrol (buratrol) method. A drip rate *must* be established to ensure patient safety from an overdose. A *microdrip* 60 gtt/ml or 60 ml/hr is the usual method of administering medications in critical care settings. The following problems are calculated using the microdrip.

EXAMPLE: *Doctor orders:*   Regular insulin 35 U/hr IV drip.

Have: Pharmacy has delivered 500 ml 0.9% NS with 500 U regular insulin added.

To infuse 35 U/hr, what will be the ml/hr or gtt/min rate?

ANSWER: 500 U : 500 ml : : 35 U : x ml   PROOF: $500 \times 35 = 17,500$

$500x = 500 \times 35 = 17,500$ $500 \times 35 = 17,500$

$500x = 17,500$

$x = 35$ ml/hr or 35 gtt/hr

Therefore:

$$\frac{D}{M} \times V = gtt/min$$

$$\frac{\overset{1}{\cancel{60}}}{\underset{1}{\cancel{60}}} \times 35 = 35 \text{ gtt/min}$$

6H Worksheet

1. Doctor ordered regular insulin* 35 U/hr. The IV solution label reads "200 U regular insulin in 500 ml N.S." How many drops per minute will you regulate the IV to infuse 35 U/hr?

---

*Only regular insulin can be used intravenously.

Section 6, Unit H answer sheet is on p. 130.

2. Ordered: regular insulin 12 U/hr. Pharmacy sent an IV solution containing 100 ml N.S. with 100 U regular insulin. How many gtt/min will you regulate the IV?

3. Doctor ordered 15 U regular insulin/hr. On hand is regular insulin U 100 and 250 ml IV 0.9% N.S. If you mix 100 U of insulin with 250 ml of the IV solution, how many ml/hr will deliver 15 U of medication per hour?

4. Ordered: heparin 10,000 U in 24 hr. The pharmacy sent 500 ml N.S. with 10,000 U of heparin. How many drops per minute will deliver 10,000 U in 24 hr?

5. Doctor ordered heparin 700 U/hr. Pharmacy sends 500 ml 0.9% N.S. with 10,000 U heparin. How many drops per minute will you need to calculate to administer the ordered dose?

6. Ordered: heparin 635 U/hr. Pharmacy has sent 250 ml D5W with 20,000 U heparin. How many ml/hr and gtt/min are needed to deliver 635 U/hr?

Section 6 INTRAVENOUS CALCULATIONS
ANSWER SHEETS

6B Answer sheet

KNOW: **1** $\dfrac{TV^*}{TT}$ = ml/hr

2 $\dfrac{D^*}{M} \times V$ = gtt/min

1. *Step 1:* $\dfrac{TV}{TT} = \dfrac{1000}{8} = 125$ ml/hr

   Step 2: $\dfrac{10}{60} \times \dfrac{125 \text{ ml}}{1} = \dfrac{1}{6} \times \dfrac{125}{1} = \dfrac{125}{6} = 20.8 = 21$ gtt/min

2. *Step 2:* $\dfrac{12}{60} \times \dfrac{200}{1} = \dfrac{1}{5} \times \dfrac{200}{1} = \dfrac{200}{5} = 40$ gtt/min

3. *Step 2:* $\dfrac{10}{30} \times \dfrac{100}{1} = \dfrac{1}{3} \times \dfrac{100}{1} = \dfrac{100}{3} = 33.3$ or 33 gtt/min

4. *Step 1:* $\dfrac{1500}{12} = 125$ ml/hr

   Step 2: $\dfrac{15}{60} \times \dfrac{125}{1} = \dfrac{1}{4} \times \dfrac{125}{1} = 31.2$ or 31 gtt/min

5. *Step 2:* $\dfrac{60}{60} \times \dfrac{50}{1} = \dfrac{1}{1} \times \dfrac{50}{1} = \dfrac{50}{1} = 50$ gtt/min

---

*Always reduce fraction *before* multiplying.

6. *Step 1:* $\dfrac{1500}{8} = 188$ ml/hr

    Step 2: a. $\dfrac{10}{60} \times \dfrac{188}{1} = \dfrac{1}{6} \times \dfrac{188}{1} = \dfrac{188}{6} = 31.2$ or 31 gtt/min

            b. $\dfrac{13}{60} \times \dfrac{188}{1} = \dfrac{2444}{60} = 40.7$ or 41 gtt/min

7. *Step 2:* $\dfrac{10}{45} \times \dfrac{75}{1} = \dfrac{750}{45} = 16.6$ or 17 gtt/min

6C Answer sheet

$\dfrac{\text{Total volume}}{\text{Total time}} = $ ml/hr

$\dfrac{\text{Drop factor}}{\text{Time (min)}} \times \text{V/hr} = $ gtt/min

1. *Step 1:* $\dfrac{TV}{TT} = \dfrac{2000}{24} = 83.3$ ml/hr

2. *Step 1:* $\dfrac{TV}{TT} = \dfrac{1500}{8} = 187.5 = 188$ ml/hr

    Step 2: $\dfrac{15}{60} \times \dfrac{188}{1} = \dfrac{\overset{1}{\cancel{15}}}{\underset{4}{\cancel{60}}} \times \dfrac{188}{1} = 47$ gtt/min

3. *Step 1:* $\dfrac{TV}{TT} = \dfrac{3000}{24} = 125$ ml/hr

    Step 2: $\dfrac{60}{60} \times \dfrac{125}{1} = 1 \times 125 = 125$ gtt/min

4. *Step 1:* $\dfrac{TV}{TT} = \dfrac{500}{4} = 125$ ml/hr

    Step 2: $\dfrac{13}{\underset{12}{\cancel{60}}} \times \dfrac{\overset{25}{\cancel{125}}}{1} = 27.08$ or 27 gtt/min

5. *Step 1:* $\dfrac{TV}{TT} = \dfrac{1000}{12} = 83.3 = 83$ ml/hr

   Step 2: $\dfrac{\overset{1}{\cancel{60}}}{\underset{1}{\cancel{60}}} \times \dfrac{83}{1} = \dfrac{83}{1} = 83$ gtt/min

6. Start with step 2 because we already know how many ml per 30 min.

   $\dfrac{12}{\underset{3}{\cancel{30}}} \times \dfrac{\overset{10}{\cancel{100}}}{1} = \dfrac{120}{3} = 40$ gtt/min

7. *Step 1:* $\dfrac{TV}{TT} = \dfrac{2000}{24} = 83.3 = 83$ ml/hr

   Step 2: $\dfrac{15}{60} \times \dfrac{83}{1} = \dfrac{\overset{1}{\cancel{15}}}{\underset{4}{\cancel{60}}} \times \dfrac{83}{1} = \dfrac{83}{4} = 20.75 = 21$ gtt/min

8. *Step 1:* $\dfrac{TV}{TT} = \dfrac{150}{10} = 15$ ml/hr

   Step 2: $\dfrac{\overset{1}{\cancel{60}}}{\underset{1}{\cancel{60}}} \times \dfrac{15}{1} = 15$ gtt/min

9. *Step 1:* $\dfrac{TV}{TT} = \dfrac{1500}{12} = 125$ ml/hr

   Step 2: $\dfrac{\overset{1}{\cancel{15}}}{\underset{4}{\cancel{60}}} \times \dfrac{125}{1} = \dfrac{125}{4} = 31$ gtt/min

10. MEMORIZE: $\dfrac{TV}{TT} = $ ml/hr

    $\dfrac{\text{Drop factor}}{\text{Time (min)}} \times V/hr = $ gtt/min or $\dfrac{D}{M} \times V = $ gtt/min

6D Answer sheet

REMEMBER: *Step 1:* $\dfrac{TV}{TT} = $ ml/hr

Step 2: $\dfrac{D}{M} \times V = $ gtt/min

1. *Step 2:* $\dfrac{1\cancel{0}}{6\cancel{0}} \times 100 = \dfrac{100}{6} = 16.6 = 17$ gtt/min

2. *Step 1:* $\dfrac{TV}{TT} = \dfrac{1000}{6} = 166.6 = 167$ ml/hr

 Step 2: $\dfrac{15}{60} \times \dfrac{167}{1} = \dfrac{\overset{1}{\cancel{15}}}{\underset{4}{\cancel{60}}} \times \dfrac{167}{1} = \dfrac{167}{4} = 41.57 = 42$ gtt/min

3. *Step 2:* $\dfrac{10}{30} \times \dfrac{50}{1} = \dfrac{1\cancel{0}}{3\cancel{0}} \times \dfrac{50}{1} = \dfrac{50}{3} = 16.6 = 17$ gtt/min

4. *Step 2:* $\dfrac{60}{60} \times \dfrac{100}{1} = \dfrac{\overset{1}{\cancel{60}}}{\underset{1}{\cancel{60}}} \times \dfrac{100}{1} = 100$ gtt/min

5. *Step 1:* $\dfrac{TV}{TT} = \dfrac{2000}{12} = 166.6 = 167$ ml/hr

 Step 2: $\dfrac{60}{60} \times \dfrac{167}{1} = \dfrac{\overset{1}{\cancel{60}}}{\underset{1}{\cancel{60}}} \times \dfrac{167}{1} = 167$ gtt/min

6. *Step 2:* $\dfrac{12}{30} \times \dfrac{100}{1} = \dfrac{12}{3\cancel{0}} \times \dfrac{10\cancel{0}}{1} = \dfrac{120}{3} = 40$ gtt/min

7. *Step 1:* $\dfrac{TV}{TT} = \dfrac{1500}{24} = 62.5 = 63$ ml/hr

 Step 2: $\dfrac{10}{60} \times \dfrac{63}{1} = \dfrac{1\cancel{0}}{6\cancel{0}} \times \dfrac{63}{1} = \dfrac{63}{6} \times 10.5 = 11$ gtt/min

8. *Step 1:* $\dfrac{TV}{TT} = \dfrac{500}{8} = 62.5 = 63$ ml/hr

Step 2: $\dfrac{60}{60} \times \dfrac{63}{1} = \dfrac{\overset{1}{\cancel{60}}}{\underset{1}{\cancel{60}}} \times \dfrac{63}{1} = 63$ gtt/min

6E Answer sheet

1. $\dfrac{10}{60} \times \dfrac{100}{1} = \dfrac{1}{6} \times \dfrac{100}{1} = \dfrac{100}{6} = 16.6$ or 17 gtt/min

2. $\dfrac{15}{20} \times \dfrac{50}{1} = \dfrac{\overset{3}{\cancel{15}}}{\underset{4}{\cancel{20}}} \times \dfrac{50}{1} = \dfrac{150}{4} = 37.5$ or 38 gtt/min

3. $\dfrac{60}{30} \times \dfrac{50}{1} = \dfrac{\overset{2}{\cancel{60}}}{\underset{1}{\cancel{30}}} \times \dfrac{50}{1} = 100$ gtt/min

4. $\dfrac{12}{60} \times \dfrac{100}{1} = \dfrac{\overset{1}{\cancel{12}}}{\underset{5}{\cancel{60}}} \times \dfrac{100}{1} = \dfrac{100}{5} = 20$ gtt/min

1. DOBUTAMINE

   Step 1: lb to kg
   1 kg:2.2 lb::x kg:155 lb   PROOF: $1 \times 155 = 155$
   $2.2x = 155$ $2.2 \times 70.4 = 154.8$
   $x = 70.4$ kg

   Step 2: For maximum rate per minute, calculate with 10 μg/kg/min.

   Step 3: mg to μg
   1 mg:1000 μg::200 mg:x μg   PROOF: $1 \times 200,000 = 200,000$
   $x = 1000 \times 200 = 200,000$ $1000 \times 200 = 200,000$
   $x = 200,000$ μg

   Step 4: μg/kg/min
   10 μg:1 kg::x μg:70.4 kg   PROOF: $10 \times 70.4 = 704$
   $x = 10 \times 70.4 = 704$ $1 \times 704 = 704$
   $x = 704$ μg/min for 70.4 kg weight

   Step 5: min to deliver 200,000 μg
   704 μg:1 min::200,000 μg:x min   PROOF: $1 \times 200,000 = 200,000$
   $704x = 200,000$ $704 \times 284 = 199,936$
   $x = 284$ min $\div$ 60 = 4 hr and 42 min

   Step 6: 250 mg:20 ml::200 mg:x ml
   $250x = 20 \times 200 = 4000$
   $250x = 4000$
   $x = 16$ ml   Add to 50 ml of IV solution = 66 ml to be infused.

   Step 7: $\dfrac{60}{284} \times 66 = \dfrac{3960}{284} = 13.9 = 14$ gtt/min

   Step 8: The current rate of infusion is 125 ml/hr with a microdrip, which means 125 gtt/min. Therefore the IV rate must be changed to 14 gtt/min until 66 ml is infused, which will take 4 hr and 42 min.

2. QUINIDINE SULFATE
   Step 1: ml of solution = 250 mg

   Have   **Want to know**

   800 mg : 50 ml : : 250 mg : x ml

   $800x = 50 \times 250 = 12,500$

   $800x = 12,500$

   $x = 15.625 = 15.6$ ml

   PROOF: $800 \times 15.625 = 12,500$

   $50 \times 250 = 12,500$

   Step 2: min/250 mg to infuse

   Have   **Want to know**

   16 mg : 1 min : : 250 mg : x min

   $16x = 250$

   $x = 15.625 = 16$ min to infuse 250 mg quinidine

   PROOF: $16 \times 15.625 = 250$

   $1 \times 250 = 250$

   Step 3: gtt/min

   Know   **Want to know**

   60 gtt : 15.6 ml : : x gtt : 15.6 ml

   $15.6x = 60 \times 15.6 = 936$

   $15.6x = 936$

   $x = 60$ gtt/min

   PROOF: $15.6 \times 60 = 936$

   $60 \times 15.6 = 936$

   Step 4: Yes, the current IV must be adjusted to infuse at a slower rate (60 gtt/min for 16 min).

3. NITROPRUSSIDE
   Step 1: lb to kg

   Know   **Want to know**

   1 kg : 2.2 lb : : x kg : 165 lb

   $2.2x = 165$

   $x = 75$ kg

   PROOF: $2.2 \times 75 = 165$

   $1 \times 165 = 165$

   Step 2: mg to μg

   Know   **Want to know**

   1 mg : 1000 μg : : 50 mg : x μg

   $x = 1000 \times 50 = 50,000$

   $x = 50,000$ μg

   PROOF: $50 \times 1000 = 50,000$

   $1 \times 50,000 = 50,000$

Step 3: μg/kg/min

Know　　　**Want to know**

3 μg:1 kg::x μg:75 kg

x = 3 × 75 = 225

x = 225 μg/min

PROOF: 1 × 225 = 225
　　　　3 × 75 = 225

Step 4: total volume

250 ml D5W　　D5W = 253 ml

+ 3 ml/50 mg Nipride

253 ml-total volume to be infused

Step 5: μg/min

Know　　　**Want to know**

225 μg:1 min::50,000 μg:x min

225x = 50,000

x = 222.2 min ÷ 60 = 3 hr and 42 min

PROOF: 1 × 50,000 = 50,000
　　　　225 × 222.2 = 49,995

Step 6: gtt/min

$$\frac{60}{222} \times 253 = \frac{15,180}{222} = 68.3 = 68 \text{ gtt/min}$$

Step 7: The current rate of infusion is 85 ml/hr or 85 gtt/min. The rate for nitroprusside is 68 gtt/min; therefore the rate has to be decreased for 3 hr and 42 min.

4. LIDOCAINE

Step 1: lb to kg

Know　　**Want to know**

1 kg:2.2 lb::x kg:182

2.2x = 182

x = 82.7 kg

PROOF: 2.2 × 82.7 = 181.9
　　　　1 × 182 = 182

Step 2: maximum dose for patient using μg and mg/min

Know　　　**Want to know**

50 μg:1 kg::x μg:82.7 kg

x = 50 × 82.7 = 4135

x = 4135 μg/min for patient weighing 82.7 kg

4.1 mg/min for patient weighing 82.7 kg

Therefore 4.0 mg/min order is safe.

PROOF: 1 × 4135 = 4135
　　　　50 × 82.7 = 4135

Step 3: mg/min (hr)   Is this a safe dose for 1 hr?

Know   **Want to know**

4 mg:1 min::x mg:60 min

$x = 4 \times 60 = 240$

$x = 240$ mg/hr

PROOF: $1 \times 240 = 240$
$4 \times 60 = 240$

This is a safe dose for patient. Literature states no more than 300 mg over a 1 hr period.

Step 4: μg or mg or g/ml

Know   **Want to know**

1 g:1000 ml::x g:1 ml

$1000x = 1$

$x = 0.001$ g in 1 ml = 1 mg/ml = 1000 μg/ml

PROOF: $1 \times 1 = 1$
$1000 \times 0.001 = 1$

Step 5: ml/hr

Know   **Want to know**

1 mg:1 ml::240 mg:x ml

$x = 240$ ml/hr = 240 gtt/min (microdrip)

Change existing IV rate from 100 ml/hr to 240 ml/hr

PROOF: $1 \times 240 = 240$
$1 \times 240 = 240$

6H Answer sheet _____

1. **Know**   **Want to know**

   $200 \text{ U}:500 \text{ ml}::35 \text{ U}:x \text{ ml}$

   $200x = 500 \times 35 = 17{,}500$

   $200x = 17{,}500$

   $x = 87.5 = 88 \text{ ml/hr or gtt/min}$

   PROOF: $200 \times 87.5 = 17{,}500$

            $500 \times 35 = 17{,}500$

2. $100 \text{ ml}:100 \text{ U}::x \text{ ml}:12 \text{ U}$

   $100x = 100 \times 12 = 1200$

   $100x = 1200$

   $x = 12 \text{ ml or } 12 \text{ gtt/min}$

   PROOF: $100 \times 12 = 1200$

            $100 \times 12 = 1200$

3. **Know**   **Want to know**

   $250 \text{ ml}:100 \text{ U}::x \text{ ml}:15 \text{ U}$

   $100x = 250 \times 15 = 3750$

   $100x = 3750$

   $x = 37.5 = 38 \text{ ml/hr or } 38 \text{ gtt/min}$

   PROOF: $100 \times 37.5 = 3750$

            $250 \times 15 = 3750$

4. $\dfrac{60}{1440 \text{ } (24 \text{ hr} \times 60 \text{ min})} \times 500 = \dfrac{2500}{120} = 20.8 = 21 \text{ gtt/min}$

5. $500 \text{ ml}:10{,}000 \text{ U}::x \text{ ml}:700 \text{ U}$

   $10{,}000x = 500 \times 700 = 350{,}000$

   $10{,}000x = 350{,}000$

   $x = 35 \text{ ml/hr or gtt/min}$

   PROOF: $10{,}000 \times 35 = 350{,}000$

            $500 \times 700 = 350{,}000$

6. $250 \text{ ml}:20{,}000 \text{ U}::x \text{ ml}:635 \text{ U}$

   $20{,}000x = 250 \times 635 = 158{,}750$

   $20{,}000x = 158{,}750$

   $x = 7.9 = 8 \text{ ml/hr or } 8 \text{ gtt/min}$

   PROOF: $7.9 \times 20{,}000 = 158{,}000$

            $250 \times 635 = 158{,}750$

Section 6 INTRAVENOUS CALCULATIONS QUIZ

Write the two rules or two steps *first* and then analyze your problems. Will you begin with step 1 or step 2?

1. Doctor ordered 3000 ml for 24 hr. Drop factor is 15. How many gtt/min?

2. Ordered: 75 ml to be infused in 45 min. Drop factor is 10. How many gtt/min?

3. Doctor ordered 1000 ml to be infused in 12 hr IV. How many gtt/min if drop factor is 12?

4. Ordered: 1200 ml to be infused in 8 hr. Drop factor is microdrip. How many gtt/min?

5. You have 2000 ml 5% D/W being infused for 24 hr. Drop factor is 10. How many ml/hr?

6. You have 1500 ml NS to infuse. Drop factor is 15. Solution is to be given over a 12 hr period. How many ml/hr? _____ How many gtt/min? _____

7. You have 3000 ml 5 D/W being infused for 24 hr with 0.5 g of penicillin in each 1000 ml. Drop factor is 60, by microdrip. How many gtt/min?

8. You have 500 ml NS being infused for 6 hr. Drop factor is 13. How many gtt/min?

9. Ordered: 1000 ml to run for 12 hr on microdrip. How many gtt/min will you regulate flow?

Section 6 Intravenous calculations quiz answer sheet_____

1. 125 ml/hr
   31 gtt/min

2. 17 gtt/min

3. 83 ml/hr
   17 gtt/min

4. 150 ml/hr
   150 gtt/min

5. 83 ml/hr
   14 gtt/min

6. 125 ml/hr
   31 gtt/min

7. 125 ml/hr
   125 gtt/min

8. 83 ml/hr
   18 gtt/min

9. 83 ml/hr
   83 gt/min

SECTION 7

Solutions

Math objectives

1. *State percent of sodium chloride in normal saline solution.*
2. *Solve percent solution problem using ratio and proportion method.*

UNIT A _____

Rules

A solution consists of two parts: the solvent (usually water) and the solute (a solid, liquid, or gas) dissolved in the solvent. Solution problems are percent problems. Remember that *percentage* means hundred*ths*. A percent number is a fraction whose top number is stated and bottom number is understood to be 100.

EXAMPLE: **1** 20% is the same as $^{20}/_{100}$. To make a ratio out of a fraction all you must do is put the top number on the left and the bottom number on the right.

2 The fraction $^{20}/_{100}$ is the same as the ratio 20:100.

One ml (or cc) of water weighs 1 g. Therefore g and ml (or cc) can be used interchangeably. If the solute (part being dissolved) is a liquid, then ml (or cc) can be used. (The use of ml is preferred over cc, since cc is properly used with gases. Nevertheless cc is occasionally used in this text.) If the solute is a solid such as NaCl (salt) or tablets, then the g symbol is used.

Normal saline (isotonic sodium chloride) is 0.9%. As a ratio it is *always* written 0.9:100. Half-strength NaCl is 0.45%. As a ratio it is *always* written 0.45:100.

Percent problems for solutions

RULE: **1** Set up a ratio and proportion with what you *have* on hand on the *left* and what you *want* to make on the *right*.

EXAMPLE: Make up 250 ml of a 20% acetic acid solution.

Have   **Want**

20 ml acetic acid:100 ml water::x ml acetic acid:250 ml water

$100x = 5000$ PROOF: $100 \times 50 = 5000$

$x = 50$ ml acetic acid $20 \times 250 = 5000$

Section 7 answer sheets begin on p. 139.

When working with liquids such as acetic acid, you must *subtract* the amount of *full-strength* acetic acid needed (in this problem it is 50 ml) from the total amount of solution ordered to determine how much water to add.

RULE: **2** When you have figured out how much solvent to use, put that in the container first and fill to the amount of solution ordered.

EXAMPLE: We know we need 50 ml of full strength acetic acid. The total amount of solution (20%) ordered was 250 ml.

   250 ml ordered
   −50 ml ml full-strength acetic acid
   200 ml water added to the 50 ml of 20% acetic acid = 250 ml of 20% solution

NOTE: This ratio and proportion setup works whenever you are preparing a solution from a *full-strength* solid or liquid such as salt or 100% solutions.

RULE: **3** If the solution you are to use for the preparation of the desired solution is a ratio, just use the ratio for the *have* side or *left* side of equation.

EXAMPLE: Make up 1 pint of a 1:1000 Zephiran Chloride solution.

Have   **Want**

1 g:1000 ml::x g:500 ml
1000x = 500
x = 0.5 g

You will measure $\frac{1}{2}$ g or ml of 1:1000 Zephiran Chloride solution and pour it into 499.5 ml of water = 500 ml of 1:1000 solution.

RULE: **4** When the answer is in grams and the tablets are in grains, you must set up a ratio and proportion, using the method as in Section 5.

EXAMPLE: 1 g = gr 15

UNIT B

7B Worksheet

1. Make up 500 ml of normal saline solution. How many g of salt will you use? How many tsp. is this?

2. Make up 1000 ml of normal saline solution. How many g or tsp. of salt will you add?

3. Doctor ordered 300 ml of a 5% acetic acid solution. How much full-strength acetic acid will you use and how much water?

4. Ordered: 250 ml of a 10% acetic acid solution. How much full-strength acetic acid will you use and how much water?

5. Doctor ordered 150 ml of normal saline solution for a mouthwash. How much salt will you use? How can this problem be simplified?

6. Make up 200 ml of a 10% solution of acetic acid from full-strength liquid. How many ml of acetic acid will you use?

7. You are to prepare NS solution (0.9%) as an enema. You will use _____ tsp. of table salt in 1000 ml of H_2O.

8. You are to prepare a NS throat irrigation. You will mix _____ tsp. of salt with 500 ml H_2O.

9. You are to give $1^{1}/_{2}$% vinegar douch. The douche bag holds 1 qt. You will add _____ tsp. of vinegar to 1 qt of H_2O.

UNIT C _____

7C Worksheet _____

1. Prepare 4 L of a 1:500 ml solution of Lysol. How many ml of Lysol will you need?

2. How many 5 gr tablets must be dissolved to make 1 L of 1:500 solution?

3. Prepare 1 L of a 1:750 solution of potassium permanganate. How many g of $KMNO_4$ will you need?

4. Prepare 1 pt of a 1:750 solution of potassium permanganate. Tablets of $KMNO_4$ containing gr 1 each are on stock. How many grains or tablets will you use? Is this a one-step or a two-step problem?

Section 7 SOLUTIONS ANSWER SHEETS

7B Answer sheet

1. **Have**   **Want**

   0.9 g : 100 ml : : x g NaCl : 500 ml water

   $100x = 450$

   $x = 4.5$ g salt added to 500 ml water

   PROOF: $0.9 \times 500 = 450$

   $100 \times 4.5 = 450$

   REMEMBER: 1 tsp. = 4 to 5 ml or g

2. **Have**   **Want**

   0.9 g : 100 ml : : x g NaCl : 1000 ml water

   $100x = 900$

   $x = 9$ g salt, or add 2 tsp. of salt

   PROOF: $0.9 \times 1000 = 900$

   $9 \times 100 = 900$

   REMEMBER: When normal saline is ordered, make up 500 ml using 1 tsp. salt. If you need only enough for a throat gargle, just discard the unused portion.

3. **Have**   **Want**

   5 ml : 100 ml : : x ml acetic acid : 300 ml water

   $100x = 1500$

   $x = 15$ ml acetic acid

   PROOF: $100 \times 15 = 1500$

   $5 \times 300 = 1500$

   Pour 15 ml of 5% acetic acid into a container. Then add water to the 300 ml mark.

     300 ml desired

   -15 ml acetic acid

     285 ml water

4. **Have**   **Want**

   10 ml : 100 ml : : x ml acetic acid : 250 ml

   $100x = 2500$

   $x = 25$ ml acetic acid

   PROOF: $10 \times 250 = 2500$

   $100 \times 25 = 2500$

   Pour 25 ml full-strength acetic acid into container. Then add water to the 250 ml mark.

     250 ml desired

   -25 ml acetic acid

     225 ml water

5. **Have**   **Want**

$\quad$ 0.9 g : 100 ml :: x g salt : 150 ml $\qquad\qquad$ PROOF: $100 \times 1.35 = 135$

$\quad$ $100x = 135$ $\qquad\qquad\qquad\qquad\qquad\qquad\qquad$ $0.9 \times 150 = 135$

$\quad$ $x = 1.35 = 1$ ml or g salt

Add 1 g of salt to 150 ml of water. Since it is difficult to measure 1 g or ml of salt, just make up a normal saline solution of 500 ml water (1 pt) and add 1 tsp. (4 to 5 ml) of salt. Discard any unused portion.

6. **Have**   **Want**

$\quad$ 10 ml : 100 ml :: x ml acetic acid : 200 ml water $\qquad$ PROOF: $100 \times 20 = 2000$

$\quad$ $100x = 2000$ $\qquad\qquad\qquad\qquad\qquad\qquad\qquad$ $10 \times 200 = 2000$

$\quad$ $x = 20$ ml acetic acid

Add 20 ml of 10% acetic acid to the container; add water to make 200 ml.

$\quad$ 200 ml desired

$\quad$ $\underline{-20}$ ml acetic acid

$\quad$ 180 ml water

7. **Have**   **Want**

$\quad$ 0.9 g : 100 ml :: x g NaCl : 1000 ml water $\qquad$ PROOF: $100 \times 9 = 900$

$\quad$ $100x = 900$ $\qquad\qquad\qquad\qquad\qquad\qquad\qquad$ $0.9 \times 1000 = 900$

$\quad$ $x = 9$ g NaCl or 2 tsp.

Always prepare a 1000 ml solution for an enema.

8. **Have**   **Want**

$\quad$ 0.9 g : 100 ml :: x g NaCl : 500 ml water $\qquad$ PROOF: $100 \times 4.5 = 450$

$\quad$ $100x = 450$ $\qquad\qquad\qquad\qquad\qquad\qquad\qquad$ $0.9 \times 500 = 450$

$\quad$ $x = 4.5$ g salt $= 1$ tsp.

You should have this problem memorized by now. REMEMBER: 1 teaspoon in 1 pint of water gives 500 ml of normal saline solution.

9. **Have**   **Want**

$\quad$ $1^{1}/_{2}$ ml : 100 ml :: x ml vinegar : 1000 ml $\qquad$ PROOF: $100 \times 15 = 1500$

$\quad$ $100x = {}^{3}/_{2} = {}^{1000}/_{1} = 1500$ $\qquad\qquad\qquad\qquad$ $1^{1}/_{2} \times 1000 = 1500$

$\quad$ $100x = 1500$

$\quad$ $x = 15$ ml vinegar

Add 15 ml or 3 tsp. of vinegar to the 1 L container. Add 985 ml water to make up 1000 ml of solution.

7C Answer sheet

1. **Have**   **Want**

   1 ml : 500 ml : : x ml : 4000 ml   PROOF: $500 \times 8 = 4000$

   $500x = 4000$ $1 \times 4000 = 4000$

   $x = 8$ ml Lysol

   Pour   8 ml Lysol

   Add   <u>3992</u> ml water

                 4000 ml of a 1 : 500 solution of Lysol

2. **Have**   **Want**

   1 g : 500 ml : : x g : 1000 ml   PROOF: $500 \times 2 = 1000$

   $500x = 1000$ $1 \times 1000 = 1000$

   $x = 2$ g

   Now grams must be changed to grains.

   Know   **Want**

   1 g : gr 15 : : 2 g : gr x PROOF: $15 \times 2 = 30$

   $1x = 30$ $1 \times 30 = 30$

   $x = 30$ gr

   This means dissolve gr 30 (or six 5-grain tablets) in 1000 ml of water to make 1000 ml of a 1 : 500 solution.

3. **Have**   **Want**

   1 g : 750 ml : : x g : 1000 ml   PROOF: $750 \times 1.33^{1}/_{3} = 1000$

   $750x = 1000$ $1 \times 1000 = 1000$

   $x = 1.33^{1}/_{3}$ g

   Pour 1.3 ml $KMNO_4$ full strength. Add 998.7 ml water to make 1000.00 ml = 1 : 750 solution.

4. **Have**   **Want**

   1 g : 750 ml : : x g : 500 ml   PROOF: $750 \times 0.66^{2}/_{3} = 500$

   $750x = 500$ $1 \times 500 = 500$

   $x = 0.66^{2}/_{3}$ g $= 0.7$ g

   Now grams must be changed to grains.

   Know   **Want**

   1 g : gr 15 : : 0.7 g : gr x PROOF: $15 \times 0.7 = 10.5$

   $1x = 15 \times 0.7 = 10.5$ $1 \times 10.5 = 10.5$

   $x = $ gr 10.5

   Each tablet of $KMNO_4$ contains 1 grain. Dissolve $10^{1}/_{2}$ tablets of $KMNO_4$ (1 grain each) in 500 ml water to make 500 ml of 1 : 750 solution.

141

SECTION 8

Medications from powder and crystals

Math objectives

1. *Given multidose antibiotic vial and doctor's order for specified amount, calculate milliliter to be administered.*

2. *Given multidose vial with various dilutions to make, determine best strength to mix for designated order.*

UNIT A

Explanation

Diluting powder or crystals in vials

Directions for dissolving drugs in vials can be found in the accompanying literature. Information given will be the volume of the powder after it is dissolved in NS or distilled water. For instance, the directions may read: "Add 1.4 ml NS to make 2 ml of reconstituted solution." These directions tell the user that the powder takes up 0.6 ml of space.

$$1.4 \text{ ml} + 0.6 \text{ ml} = 2 \text{ ml}$$

Next read the literature to find out how many units, grams, milligrams, and so on, are in each milliliter of the reconstituted drug. This is where the ratio and proportion problem begins.

EXAMPLE: DIRECTIONS: Add 1.4 ml distilled water (sterile) to make 600,000 units of penicillin per 2 ml.

Doctor ordered 300,000 U penicillin IM q.6h.

Have	**Want**	
2 ml : 600,000 U : : x ml : 300,000 U		PROOF: $2 \times 3 = 6$
$6x = 6$		$6 \times 1 = 6$
$x = 1$ ml		

Give 1 ml of reconstituted solution for each 300,000 U.

Always label vial according to amount of units per milliliter.

EXAMPLE: 300,000 U/ml, date, initials.

Many solutions are unstable after being reconstituted. Read directions carefully for storing in refrigerator or in a dark place. There is usually a time limit or expiration date on vial. It is important to date, label, and initial all reconstituted medications.

Section 8 answer sheets begin on p. 147.

UNIT B

8B Worksheet

1. Doctor ordered Prostaphlin (sodium oxacillin) 500 mg IM. You have a multidose vial that reads: "Prostaphlin; add 5.7 ml sterile water for injection." Each 1.5 ml of solution contains 0.25 g. How many ml will you give?

2. Ordered: potassium penicillin G (Pfizerpen) 300,000 units IM. You have a multidose vial containing 1 million units and the following directions:

Ml of diluent added	Units per ml
19.6	50,000
9.6	100,000
3.6	250,000
1.6	500,000

Which dilution will you make and label? How many ml or part of ml will you give?

3. Doctor ordered 200 mg Keflin IM q.4h. Available is Keflin (cephalothin sodium) 1 g in a 10 ml vial. Each g of Keflin should be diluted with 4 ml of sterile water for injection. The reconstituted material will provide two 500 mg doses of 2.2 ml each. How many ml will you give?

4. Ordered: 125 mg Kefazol (cefazolin sodium) IM. Available is cefazolin sodium 500 mg with the following directions for reconstitution: "Add 2 ml sterile water for injection or 0.9% sodium chloride for injection. Provides approximate volume of 2.2 ml (225 mg/ml) after reconstitution. Store in refrigerator. Protect from light, and use within 96 hours. If kept at room temperature, use within 24 hours." How many ml will you give?

5. Doctor ordered Totacillin-N (sodium ampicillin) 500 mg IM stat. Available is a powdered form labeled "0.50 g for IV or IM use. For IM use, add at least 1.7 ml sterile water for injection, U.S.P. Use solution within 1 hr after reconstituting." Each ml will contain 0.25 g. How many ml will you give?

6. Ordered: Achromycin V 500 mg IV volutrol stat. Available is Achromycin (tetracycline hydrochloride) 0.50 g for IV administration only. Directions: "Add 10 ml of sterile water for injection. After solution has been prepared, it should be further diluted prior to administration to at least 100 ml (up to 1000 ml)." How many ml will you dilute in the IV volutrol bag, which holds 100 ml?

7. Doctor ordered Kantrex (kanamycin sulfate) 300 mg IM. Directions on bottle read: "Add 2.7 ml sterile water for injection to make 1 g per 3 ml." After reconstitution, how many ml will you give?

UNIT C

8C Worksheet

1. Doctor ordered penicillin G 300,000 U IM q.4h. Pharmacy sent a vial with 3,000,000 U penicillin G in dry crystal form. Directions were to dilute with 4.2 ml NS to make 5 ml. After dilution, the vial contains 5 ml per 3,000,000 U. How many ml will you give?

2. Ordered: Keflin 0.5 g IM q.6h. Pharmacy sent a vial of sodium cephalothin (Keflin) 1 g in powder form. Directions read: ''Add 4 ml sterile water to make two 0.5 g doses of 2.2 ml each.'' How many ml will you give?

3. Dilute a vial containing 500,000 U of Polycillin (ampicillin) so that each ml contains 50,000 U. How much distilled water will you need to add to the vial to get 50,000 U/ml?

4. A vial contains 1 million units of carbenicillin. Prepare the dry powder to contain a solution of 250,000 U/ml. How much distilled water will you need to add to the vial?

5. Doctor ordered 400,000 U Keflin. You have a vial with 600,000 U/ml. How many ml will you give?

6. Ordered: 1.2 million units of penicillin. You have a 10 ml vial containing 0.5 million U/ml. How many ml will you give? How many ml will be left in the vial? And how many units of penicillin will be left in the vial?

7. A vial of penicillin contains 5 million units. Doctor ordered 500,000 U. You wish to make each ml equal 500,000 U. How many ml of diluent will you use?

8. A vial is labeled ''500,000 U/ml.'' Doctor ordered 800,000 U IM q.4h. How many ml will you give?

Section 8 MEDICATIONS FROM POWDER AND CRYSTALS ANSWER SHEETS

8B Answer sheet

1. **Know**   **Want**

   1 g : 1000 mg :: x g : 500 mg   PROOF: $1000 \times 0.5 = 500$
   $1000x = 500$ $1 \times 500 = 500$
   $x = 0.5$ g

   Have   **Want**

   0.25 g : 1.5 ml :: 0.5 g : x ml   PROOF: $1.5 \times 0.5 = 0.75$
   $0.25x = 1.5 \times 0.5 = 0.75$ $0.25 \times 3 = 0.75$
   $x = 3$ ml

2. Make the 500,000 U per ml solution.

   Have   **Want**

   ~~500,000~~ U : 1 ml :: ~~300,000~~ U : x ml   PROOF: $1 \times 3 = 3$
   $5x = 3$ $5 \times 0.6 = 3$
   $x = 0.6$ ml

3. **Have**   **Want**

   500 ml : 2.2 ml :: 200 mg : x ml   PROOF: $500 \times 0.88 = 440$
   $500x = 2.2 \times 200 = 440$ $2.2 \times 200 = 440$
   $x = 0.88 = 0.9$ ml

4. **Have**   **Want**

   1 ml : 225 mg :: x ml : 125 mg   PROOF: $1 \times 125 = 125$
   $225x = 125$ $225 \times 0.55 = 123.75$
   $x = 0.55 = 0.6$ ml

5. Now that you know how to move the decimal three places to the right to change g to mg, this can be a one-step problem.

Have   **Want**

$1\ ml : 250\ mg :: x\ ml : 500\ mg$ PROOF: $1 \times 500 = 500$

$250x = 500$ $250 \times 2 = 500$

$x = 2\ ml$

6. You know that 0.50 g = 500 mg. Therefore dilute the entire vial of powder with 10 ml of sterile water for injection. Fill Volutrol with 90 ml of IV solution and add the 10 ml of reconstituted medication.

7. You know that 1 g = 1000 mg. Therefore this can be a one-step problem.

Have   **Want**

$1000\ mg : 3\ ml :: 300\ mg : x\ ml$ PROOF: $3 \times 300 = 900$

$1000x = 900$ $1000 \times 0.9 = 900$

$x = 0.9\ ml$

8C Answer sheet

1. **Have**   **Want**

   $5\ ml : 3{,}000{,}000\ U :: x\ ml : 300{,}000\ U$ PROOF: $30 \times 0.5 = 15$

   $30x = 15$ $5 \times 3 = 15$

   $x = 0.5\ ml$

   You may cross out zeros in equal amounts on both sides of the equation.

2. After diluting with 4 ml of sterile water, give 2.2 ml.

3. **Know**   **Want**

   $50{,}000\ U : 1\ ml :: 500{,}000\ U : x\ ml$ PROOF: $5 \times 10 = 50$

   $5x = 50$ $1 \times 50 = 50$

   $x = 10\ ml$

   Add 10 ml of distilled water to a vial to make 50,000 U/ml. Label vial: date, time, and U/ml.

4. **Know**   **Want**

   $250{,}000\ U : 1\ ml :: 1{,}000{,}000\ U : x\ ml$ PROOF: $25 \times 4 = 100$

   $25x = 100$ $1 \times 100 = 100$

   $x = 4\ ml$ distilled water to vial

   Each ml of carbenicillin will contain 250,000 units. Label vial: date, time, and units per ml.

5. **Have**   **Want**

    600,000 U:1 ml::400,000 U:x ml   PROOF: $1 \times 4 = 4$

    $6x = 4$ $0.6^{2}/_{3} \times 6 = 4$

    $x = 0.6^{2}/_{3} = 0.7$ ml

6. **Know**   **Want**

    500,000 U:1 ml::1,200,000 U:x ml   PROOF: $1 \times 12 = 12$

    $5x = 12$ $2.4 \times 5 = 12$

    $x = 2.4$ ml will contain 1.2 million units of penicillin

How many ml will be left in the vial?

Vial contains   10.0 ml

Gave   2.4 ml

               7.6 ml remaining in vial

How many units of penicillin will be left in the vial?

Know   **Want**

500,000 U:1 ml::x U:10 ml   PROOF: $1 \times 5,000,000 = 5,000,000$

$1x = 10 \times 500,000 = 5,000,000$ $10 \times 500,000 = 5,000,000$

$x = 5$ million units in entire vial

    5,000,000 units in entire vial

$-$ 1,200,000 units given in 2.4 ml

    3,800,000 units left in vial

7. **Have**   **Want**

    500,000 U:1 ml::5,000,000 U:x ml   PROOF: $5 \times 10 = 50$

    $5x = 50$ $1 \times 50 = 50$

    $x = 10$ ml diluent needed to make 500,000 U/ml

8. **Have**   **Want**

    500,000 U:1 ml::800,000 U:x ml   PROOF: $1 \times 8 = 8$

    $5x = 8$ $5 \times 1.6 = 8$

    $x = 1.6$ ml

SECTION 9

Insulin

Math objective

Convert insulin units to hundredths or tenths of a milliliter.

UNIT A

Explanation

The value and purity of drugs from animal sources vary. Therefore some hormones, such as insulin and heparin, are supplied in *units* (U), a standardized measurement based on strength rather than weight. You already know that insulin is an aqueous solution of the active principle hormone of the pancreas. It affects the metabolism of glucose. Insulin comes from animal sources of beef or pork pancreas.

Facts to remember

1. Insulin is supplied in units and should be given with special syringes.
2. Most commonly insulin is supplied in 10 ml vials labeled "U 100," which means 100 U/ml.
3. Insulin is also occasionally supplied in 10 ml vials labeled "U 40" (meaning 40 U/ml) or, for persons who have severe problems, "U 500" (meaning 500 U/ml).*
4. Why the three different strengths? Although you will find U 100 vials most frequently used in the hospitals, some patients have to take only a small number of units daily, such as 5 U, whereas others must take very large amounts, such as 100 U. The patients who prepare the smaller amount may find it easier to read the correct amount on a syringe calibrated for 40 U/ml and may be used to that type of syringe. The more concentrated solution of 500 U/ml is available so that people who need large amounts of insulin will receive it in *less fluid*, thus avoiding the pain of large fluid injections given frequently.
5. Insulin syringes are usually supplied in 1 ml and 0.5 ml sizes for 100 U/ml or 50 U/0.5 ml for the U 100 insulin strength. The 50 U syringe is for smaller dosages; the calibrations are larger and easier to read.

---

*U 80 is no longer available.

Section 9 answer sheets begin on p. 157.

6. What kind of order does the doctor write?

   a. The *name* of the insulin: regular, lente, NPH, etc.

   b. The *number* of units the patient will receive: regular insulin 10 U.

   c. The *time* to be given: regular insulin 10 U, in AM, ½ hr a.c.

   d. The *strength* to be given: regular insulin U 100, 10 U, in AM, ½ hr a.c.

Important rules

- If you use U 100 strength, you must use the U 100 bottle and the U 100 syringe. *Always match bottle and syringe.* If you use U 40, use the U 40 bottle and U 40 syringe.
- If there are no syringes to correspond to the same type of insulin, then use a tuberculin syringe or skin-testing syringe and, using ratio and proportion, convert your doctor's order from units to hundredths of a ml.

EXAMPLE: Doctor ordered regular insulin U 100, 30 U in AM ½ hour before meals. There are no U 100 syringes. Use ratio and proportion: You know that U 100 has 100 U in 1 ml.*

Have   **Want**

100 U : 1 ml : : 30 U : x ml

$$\frac{100x}{100} = \frac{1 \times 30}{100} = \frac{30}{100} = \frac{3}{10}$$

$x = 0.3$ ml of U 100 insulin

PROOF: $100 \times 0.3 = 30$
$1 \times 30 = 30$

Types of insulin

Short-acting (peaks first shift)

   1. Regular

   2. Semilente

Intermediate-acting (peaks second shift)

   1. NPH (neutral protamine)

   2. Lente

   3. Globin

Long-acting (peaks third shift)

   1. PZI (protamine zinc insulin)

   2. Ultralente

---

*Tuberculin syringes are calibrated in hundredths and tenths.

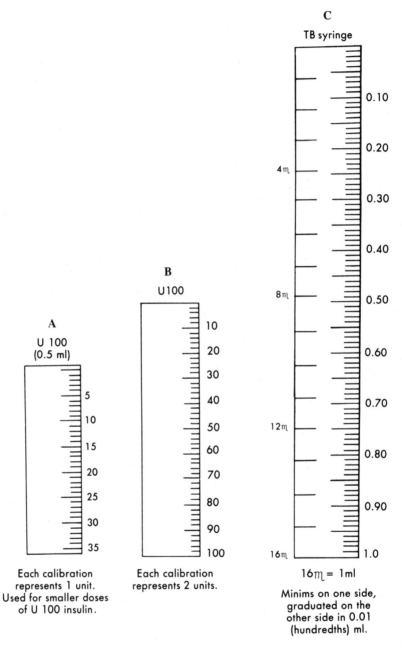

Fig. 1. A, Each calibration represents 1 unit. Used for smaller doses of U100 insulin. **B,** Each calibration represents 2 units. **C,** Minims on one side and graduated on the other side in 0.01 (hundredths) ml.

UNIT B

Types of insulin syringes

If the concentration of the insulin corresponds with the syringe, then the correct dosage of insulin can be measured directly.

EXAMPLE: Give 30 units of U 40 insulin using a U 40 syringe. Fill syringe to the 30 U calibration. Always have another registered nurse check the order, label, and dosage before administering. For U 500, have *two* nurses check.

UNIT C

9C Worksheet

Carry out to two decimal places (hundredths):

1. Convert 5 units of U 40 to ml.

2. Convert 75 units of U 100 to ml.

3. Convert 150 units of U 500 to ml.

4. Convert 45 units of U 100 to ml.

5. Doctor orders regular insulin U 40 daily in AM. What is the matter with this order?

6. Doctor orders lente insulin porcine U 100 q.AM. (*Porcine* means insulin is from pork pancreas, and bottle is labeled that way.) What would you question about this order, though?

7. If the doctor ordered NPH 100 units of insulin daily in AM, how many ml would your patient need if you used U 100 insulin?

UNIT D

9D Worksheet

Carry out to two decimal places (hundredths):

1. You are to give 35 units of regular insulin. You have a bottle labeled "regular insulin U 40" and a 1 ml tuberculin syringe. How many ml will you give?

2. Ordered: 20 units of regular insulin a.c. t.i.d.
   On hand: regular insulin U 100

   How many ml would you give? _____

3. Ordered: PZI 45 units q.d.
   On hand: PZI U 100.
   How many ml will you give? _____

4. Ordered: regular insulin 65 units.
   Available: regular insulin U 100 containing 100 U/ml.
   How many ml will you give? _____

5. Ordered: 20 units of regular insulin stat.
   Available: 40 units and 100 units of regular insulin.
   You will give either _____ ml of U 100 or _____ ml of U 40.

6. Ordered: NPH insulin 40 units SC every AM ½ hr a.c.
   Available: NPH insulin U 100.
   How many ml will you give? _____

7. Ordered: regular insulin 160 units.
   Available: regular insulin U 500.
   You will give _____ ml.

Section 9 INSULIN ANSWER SHEETS

9C Answer sheet

1. **Know**   **Want**
   40 U:1 ml::5 U:x ml   PROOF: $1 \times 5 = 5$
   $40x = 5$ $40 \times 0.12 = 4.8 = 5$
   $x = 0.12$ ml   Use a tuberculin syringe.

2. **Know**   **Want**
   100 U:1 ml::75 U:x ml   PROOF: $100 \times 0.75 = 75$
   $100x = 75$ $1 \times 75 = 75$
   $x = 0.75$ ml

3. 500 U:1 ml::150 U:x ml   PROOF: $500 \times 0.3 = 150$
   $500x = 150$ $1 \times 150 = 150$
   $x = 0.3$ ml

4. 100 U:1 ml::45 U:x ml   PROOF: $100 \times .45 = 45$
   $100x = 45$ $1 \times 45 = 45$
   $x = 0.45$ ml

5. It does not state the *amount* of U 40 insulin to be given.

6. It does not state the *amount* of U 100 insulin to be given.

7. **Know**   **Want**
   100 U:1 ml::100 U:x ml   PROOF: $100 \times 1 = 100$
   $100x = 100$ $1 \times 100 = 100$
   $x = 1$ ml

9D Answer sheet

1. **Know** **Want**

    40 U:1 ml::35 U:x ml

    $40x = 35$

    $x = 0.87$ ml

    PROOF: $40 \times 0.87 = 34.8 = 35$

    $1 \times 35 = 35$

2. **Know** **Want**

    100 U:1 ml::20 U:x ml

    $100x = 20$

    $x = 0.2$ ml

    PROOF: $100 \times 0.2 = 20$

    $1 \times 20 = 20$

3. **Know** **Want**

    100 U:1 ml::45 U:x ml

    $100x = 45$

    $x = 0.45$ ml

    PROOF: $100 \times 0.45 = 45$

    $1 \times 45 = 45$

4. **Know** **Want**

    100 U:1 ml::65 U:x ml

    $100x = 65$

    $x = 0.65$ ml

    PROOF: $100 \times 1 = 100$

    $1 \times 100 = 100$

5. **Know** **Want**

    a. 100 U:1 ml::20 U:x ml

    $100x = 20$

    $x = 0.2$ ml

    PROOF: $100 \times 0.2 = 20$

    $1 \times 20 = 20$

    Know **Want**

    b. 40 U:1 ml::20 U:x ml

    $40x = 20$

    $x = 0.5$ ml

    PROOF: $40 \times 0.5 = 20$

    $1 \times 20 = 20$

6. **Know** **Want**

    100 U:1 ml::40 U:x ml

    $100x = 40$

    $x = 0.4$ ml

    PROOF: $1 \times 40 = 40$

    $100 \times 0.4 = 40$

7. **Know** **Want**

    500 U:1 ml::160 U:x ml

    $500x = 160$

    $x = 0.32$ ml

    PROOF: $500 \times 0.32 = 160$

    $1 \times 160 = 160$

Section 9 INSULIN QUIZ

Carry out to 2 decimal places (hundredths):

1. Ordered: regular insulin 65 units deep SC stat.
   Available: regular insulin U 100 and no insulin syringe. How many ml will you give?

2. Ordered: regular insulin 4 units a.c., q.AM.
   Available: regular insulin U 40 and no insulin syringe. How many ml will you give?

3. Ordered: regular insulin 16 units with NPH insulin 30 units a.c. q.AM.
   Available: regular insulin U 100 and NPH insulin U 100 and no insulin syringes.

   a. How many ml of regular insulin will you give?

   b. How many ml of NPH will you give?

4. Ordered: lente insulin 18 U q.d.
   Available: lente insulin U 40 and no insulin syringes.

Section 9 Insulin quiz answer sheet _____

1. $x = 0.6$ ml with a tuberculin syringe

2. $x = 0.1$ ml with a tuberculin syringe

3. a. Give 0.16 ml regular insulin with a U 100 syringe.

   b. Give 0.3 ml NPH insulin with a U 100 syringe. Check literature to determine if the two can be combined in same syringe.

4. $x = 0.45$ ml with a tuberculin syringe

SECTION 10

Heparin

Math objective

Convert heparin units to hundredths or tenths of a milliliter.

UNIT A

Explanation

Sodium heparin injection, U.S.P., is a drug used to interrupt the clotting process. It may be given in therapeutic dosages or in small diluted dosages to maintain the patency of IV or IA lines. Since it is inactive orally, sodium heparin is usually administered intravenously or subcutaneously. If administered intramuscularly, the drug produces a high level of pain and may cause hematomas. Sodium heparin is obtained commercially from domestic animals slaughtered for food. The orders for heparin are highly individualized and based upon laboratory studies. Heparin comes in various strengths; so check the vial carefully before administration. Heparin is fast acting and may be counteracted with protamine sulfate. Check laboratory values for clotting times *before* administering heparin. Heparin orders, dosage, vial, and amount in syringe should be checked with another R.N.

Heparin is supplied in units, as is insulin, because the purity varies among sources. Heparin is often supplied in preprepared syringes. If you need to give less than the amount in the syringe, calculate the fractional amount you need to give and then transfer the heparin to a new syringe.*

EXAMPLE: Doctor ordered heparin 3500 U. On hand is a prepared vial containing 5000 U/ml. How many ml will you give?

Have   **Want**

$5000 \text{ U} : 1 \text{ ml} :: 3500 \text{ U} : x \text{ ml}$

$5000x = 3500$

$x = 0.7 \text{ ml}$ Use a 1 ml syringe.

---

*The new syringe with sterile needle is advisable because the heparin inside the original needle may track through the subcutaneous tissue on insertion and cause bruising. Add 0.2 ml of air to syringe to ensure that all medication is administered, which will prevent tracking.

Section 10 answer sheet is on p. 163.

UNIT B

10B Worksheet

Label and prove (carry out to nearest hundredths):

1. Give heparin 7000 U. On hand you have heparin 10,000 U/ml. How many ml will you give?
   _____

2. Ordered: 15,000 U heparin. How many ml will you give if you have heparin 20,000 U/ml?
   _____

3. Ordered: heparin 2500 U. On hand you have heparin 20,000 U/ml. How many ml will you give?

4. Ordered: heparin 17,000 U. On hand you have heparin 10,000 U/ml. How many ml will you give? _____

5. Ordered: heparin 7500 U. How many ml will you give if the vial on hand reads heparin 10,000 U/ml? _____

10B Answer sheet

1. **Have**   **Want**

   $10{,}000$ U:1 ml::$7{,}000$ U:x ml   PROOF: $1 \times 7000 = 7000$

   $10x = 7$ $10{,}000 \times 0.7 = 7000$

   $x = 0.7$ ml

2. **Have**   **Want**

   $20{,}000$ U:1 ml::$15{,}000$ U:x ml   PROOF: $1 \times 15{,}000 = 15{,}000$

   $20x = 15$ $20{,}000 \times 0.75 = 15{,}000$

   $x = 0.75$ ml

3. **Have**   **Want**

   $20{,}000$ U:1 ml::2500 U:x ml   PROOF: $200 \times 0.125 = 25$

   $200x = 25$ $1 \times 25 = 25$

   $x = 0.125 = 0.13$ ml

4. **Have**   **Want**

   $10{,}000$ U:1 ml::$17{,}000$ U:x ml   PROOF: $1 \times 17 = 17$

   $10x = 17$ $10 \times 1.7 = 17$

   $x = 1.7$ ml

5. **Have**   **Want**

   $10{,}000$ U:1 ml::7500 U:x ml   PROOF: $1 \times 75 = 75$

   $100x = 1 \times 75 = 75$ $100 \times 0.75 = 75$

   $100x = 75$

   $x = 0.75$ ml

SECTION 11

Children's dosages

Math objectives

1. *Estimate kilograms for given number of pounds.*
2. *Calculate kilograms for given number of pounds.*
3. *Calculate 24-hour dosages.*
4. *Calculate total dosage ranges in milligrams for given mg/kg formula and given weight in pounds and ounces.*
5. *Determine if pediatric drug order is within safe dosage range.*
6. *Memorize steps in mg/kg method of calculation.*
7. *Calculate pediatric dosage using BSA method.*
8. *Calculate pediatric dosage using Clark's rule.*

UNIT A _____

Explanation

Almost all medications are calculated for the average adult dosage. Babies and children receive less medication. It is extremely important for the nurse to *double check all physicians' medication orders for children and infants* to be certain that the dosage ordered is safe. Emergency situations may require quick calculations to determine the exact amount of medication to give or to determine the amount of overdose taken by the child. Remember that the nurse is legally responsible for safe dosage administration even though the physician writes the order. Prompt clarification with the physician is important if the dosage is too low to be therapeutic or too high to be safe.

There are several formulas for calculating the correct dosage for children according to age, weight, and body surface area (BSA). The formulas for weight and body surface area are more accurate and these are the methods that you will find in your references, the literature that accompanies the medication and the Physician's Desk Reference (PDR).

Mg/kg method

This method is one of the most frequently used ways to calculate safe dosage. The literature accompanying most medications states the safe amount of drug in milligrams per kilogram of body weight for a 24-hour period. The amount of mg/kg is less for children than adults. The math calculations require a determination of body weight in kilograms followed by multiplication of the weight times the mg amount permitted. The results (safe maximum limits) are compared with the physician's 24-hour order.

Section 11 answer sheets begin on p. 174.

Step 1: Estimate the child's weight in kilograms by dividing the pounds in half. (Always estimate your answers.)

Step 2: Using the ratio and proportion method, calculate the child's exact weight in kilograms to 2 decimal places. Note whether this calculation will be a one-step or two-step problem.
   a. If the child's weight is in ounces, first convert the ounces to hundredths of a pound. Add this to the pounds, which will give total weight. Then convert the pounds (total) to kilograms. (This would be a two-step calculation.)
   b. If the child's weight is already in pounds only, convert the pounds to kilograms. (This would be a one-step calculation). Is your answer close to your estimate? (This is a safety check.)

Step 3: Consult the literature* for the safe pediatric range for this medication. Multiply those amounts by the child's weight in kg. The results are the *safe* amounts of the drug allowed for the child.

Step 4: Compare the amount the physician has ordered for *24* hours with the safe amount determined by your calculations. If safe, calculate the amount of medication to be given. If unsafe, *withhold* the medication and clarify *promptly* with the physician.

EXAMPLE: Doctor ordered Lincocin 50 mg q.6h. IM. Baby weighs 12 lb, 6 oz today. On hand you have Lincocin 300 mg/ml. The literature states that the safe range is 20 mg/kg q.24h. Is this order safe? If so, how many ml will you give?

1. Weight of 12 lb, 6 oz involves a two-step conversion. It equals approximately 6 kg.

2. **Know**   **Want to know**
   a. 16 oz:1 lb::6 oz:x lb   PROOF: $16 \times 0.37 = 5.92$

   $$\frac{16x}{16} = \frac{6}{16}$$ $6 \times 1 = 6$

   Baby weighs 12.37 lb.

   b. **Know**   **Want to know**
      2.2 lb:1 kg::12.37:x kg   PROOF: $1 \times 12.37 = 12.37$

      $$\frac{2.2x}{2.2} = \frac{12.37}{2.2}$$ $2.2 \times 5.62 = 12.36$

      $x = 5.62$ kg†

---

*Use *written* literature for medication references.

†Calculate to hundredths.

3. 20 mg:1 kg::x mg:5.62 kg   PROOF: 20 × 5.62 = 112.4

    x = 20 × 5.62   1 × 112.4 = 112.4

    x = 112.4 mg (safe 24-hour dosage)

Doctor's order is 50 mg × 4 or 200 mg for 24 hours.

Safe limit for this baby is 112 mg. Hold and clarify stat.

Unsafe order.

Body surface area (BSA) method

The BSA method requires the use of a chart that has the child's weight by pounds already calculated into surface area in *square meters* (M^2). The average adult is assumed to weigh 140 lb and have 1.7 M^2 of BSA. This method can be used for children up to 12 years of age. The following is the formula to be used:

$$\frac{\text{Surface area of child in } M^2}{1.7\ M^2 \text{ (surface area of adult)}} \times \text{Average adult dose} = \text{Child's dose}$$

EXAMPLE: Child weighs 25 lb, and an adult dose of erythromycin is 500 mg IM b.i.d. How much would you administer: Use the following table:

Table 2. BSA method

Kilograms	Pounds	Surface area (square meters)	% of adult dose
1.9	4	0.15	9
2.7	6	0.20	12
4.5	10	0.24	14
6.8	15	0.36	21
9.1	20	0.42	25
11.4	25	0.52	31
13.6	30	0.60	35
18.2	40	0.70	42
22.7	50	0.84	50
27.3	60	0.98	58
31.8	70	1.10	65
36.4	80	1.20	71
40.9	90	1.32	78
45.5	100	1.40	82

$$\frac{\text{Surface area of child (M}^2) = 0.52}{\text{Surface area of adult (M}^2) = 1.7} \times 500 \text{ mg (average adult dose)}$$

Step 1: $\dfrac{0.52}{1.7} \times \dfrac{500}{1} = \dfrac{260}{1.7} = 152.9 = 153 \text{ mg}$

Step 2: Label reads "erythromycin 500 mg/2 ml."

Know   **Want**

500 mg:2 ml::153 mg:x ml   PROOF: $500 \times 0.61 = 305$

$500x = 306$ $2 \times 153 = 306$

$x = 0.61$ ml b.i.d.*

NOTE: Infants and children should receive only 0.25% to 0.40% intravenous saline solution. Electrolyte studies must be interpreted carefully for deviations from this rule. Rates should be carefully calculated and monitored with a microdrip.

Clark's rule

$$\frac{\text{Weight of child in lb}}{150 \text{ lb}} \times \text{Average adult dose} = \text{Child's dose}$$

EXAMPLE: Calculate the dose of atropine sulfate for a child weighing 40 lb. Average adult dose is 0.4 mg/ml.

Weight of child: $\dfrac{40 \text{ lb}}{150 \text{ lb}} \times 0.4 \text{ mg (average adult dose)}$

$\dfrac{40}{150} \times 0.4 = \dfrac{1.6}{15} = 0.11 \text{ mg}$

Medication available is atropine sulfate 0.4 mg/ml.

Know   **Want**

0.4 mg:1 ml::0.11 mg:x ml   PROOF: $1 \times 0.11 = 0.11$

$0.4x = 0.11$ $0.4 \times 0.27 = 0.108$

$x = 0.27$ ml*

---

*Pediatric volume less than 1 ml should be measured to hundredths in a tuberculin syringe and appropriate needle size selected.

Fried's rule

$$\frac{\text{Age in months}}{150 \text{ months}} \times \text{Average adult dose} = \text{Child's dose}$$

EXAMPLE: Calculate the dose of Valium (diazepam) for an 11-month-old baby if adult dose is 10 mg.

Age in months: $\frac{11}{150} \times 10$ mg (average adult dose)

$$\frac{11}{150} \times 10 = \frac{110}{150} = \frac{11}{15} = 0.733$$

Give 0.7 mg of Valium IM.

Available is Valium 10 mg/2 ml ampule. How many ml will you give?

Have	Want

10 mg:2 ml::0.7 mg:x ml

10x = 1.4

x = 0.14 ml

Use a tuberculin syringe and measure correct amount.

PROOF: $10 \times 0.14 = 1.4$

$2 \times 0.7 = 1.4$

Young's rule

$$\frac{\text{Age of child in years}}{\text{Age of child} + 12} \times \text{Average adult dose} = \text{Child's dose}$$

EXAMPLE: Calculate the dose of IM Polycillin if adult dose is 500 mg.

$$\frac{\text{Age}}{\text{Age} + 12} = \frac{2}{2 + 12} \times 500 \text{ mg adult dose} = \frac{2}{14} \times 500 =$$

$$\frac{1}{7} \times \frac{500}{1} = \frac{500}{7} = 71 \text{ mg}$$

Available is Polycillin 500 mg per 2 ml vial. How many ml will you give?

Have	Want

500 mg:2 ml::71 mg:x ml

500x = 142

x = 0.28 ml

PROOF: $500 \times 0.28 = 140$

$2 \times 71 = 142$

UNIT B

11B Worksheet* _____

1. Estimate the following weights in kilograms. Then convert pounds to kilograms, using ratio and proportion method. Prove your answer.
   a. 14 lb (1 step or 2 steps?)
   b. 12 lb, 2 oz (1 step or 2 steps?)
   c. 7 lb, 6 oz
   d. 15 lb, 8 oz

2. Calculate the 24-hour total dosage.
   a. 150 mg q.8h.
   b. 200 mg q.6h.
   c. 50 mg t.i.d.
   d. 75 mg q.12h.

3. Calculate the total mg/kg for safe dosage ranges for the following weights. Use ratio and proportion.
   a. 10 mg/kg   Weight is 5 kg.
   b. 5-8 mg/kg   Weight is 7.3 kg.
   c. 6-8 mg/kg   Weight is 8 lb (convert lb to kg first).
   d. 3-6 mg/kg   Weight is 5 lb, 8 oz.

*Worksheets will include only weight and BSA methods.

UNIT C

11C Worksheet*

1. Doctor ordered 10 mg phenobarbital sodium IV mg q.6h. Baby's weight today is 7 lb, 2 oz. Safe range in the literature is 3 to 6 mg/kg q.24h. On hand is phenobarbital sodium injectable 65 mg/ml. What is baby's weight in kg? What is safe dosage range for this baby? Is this order safe? If so, how many ml will you prepare for each dose?

2. The average adult dose of Garamycin (gentamicin sulfate) is 60 mg IM t.i.d. Use the BSA chart to determine how many mg would be safe to administer to a child who weighs 11.4 kg. Medication available is labeled "80 mg/2 ml vial." If safe, how many ml would you use?

3. Ordered: Garamycin IM 4 mg/kg/day divided into three doses. The child weighs 30 lb. The average adult dose is 60 mg q.8h. Use the BSA method to determine the safe individual dosage for this child. Is the doctor's order safe? If so, how many mg will the child receive in 24 hours? How many ml would the child receive in each dosage? On hand is 10 mg/ml Garamycin Pediatric Injectable.

4. Doctor ordered ampicillin 50 mg q.8h. IM. Baby weighs 5 lb, 10 oz today. Safe range for babies weighing less than 20 kg is 50 mg/kg in divided doses for 24 hours. Determine baby's weight in kg. Use the mg/kg rule to determine the safe dosage range (mg/kg) for this baby. If order is safe, calculate the correct dosage. On hand is 125 mg/5 ml Ampicillin Oral Suspension, U.S.P.

*Calculate kg to hundredths.

5. Doctor ordered Lincocin 40 mg IM b.i.d. Child weighs 9 lb, 2 oz today. Safe range for this drug is 20 mg/kg q.12h. IM. Use mg/kg method to determine if this is a safe order for the baby's weight. If so, how many ml will you give? On hand is lincomycin hydrochloride 300 mg/ml.

UNIT D

11D Worksheet* _____

1. Doctor ordered Dilantin 30 mg t.i.d. p.o. for a two-year-old child weighing 30 lb today. Safe range for this age group is 5 mg/kg/day. Use the mg/kg method to determine if this order is safe for this child. If so, how many ml will you give? On hand is Dilantin Pediatric Suspension 125 mg/5 ml.

2. Doctor ordered ampicillin 200 mg p.o. q.6h. for a baby who weighs 12 lb, 4 oz today. Safe pediatric dosage is 100 to 200 mg/kg in divided doses for 24 hr. Is this order safe? Use mg/kg method. If safe, how many ml would you give? On hand is 125 mg/5 ml Ampicillin Oral Suspension, U.S.P.

3. The average adult dose of paregoric is 8 ml p.o. Use Clark's rule to determine how many ml will be safe for a 20 lb child to receive. Round to the nearest tenth.

_____

*Calculate kg to hundredths.

4. Apomorphine hydrochloride 5 mg SC is the average adult dose. Available is apomorphine hydrochloride 10 mg/2 ml ampule. Use Clark's rule to compute the safe dosage for a 30 lb child.

5. Average adult dose of codeine sulfate is 30 mg. Use the BSA method to determine the safe dosage for a child weighing 50 lb. If the doctor ordered codeine sulfate 10 mg h.s., would it be a safe order?

Section 11 CHILDREN'S DOSAGES ANSWER SHEETS

11B Answer sheet

1. a. 14 lb = approximately 7 kg
   This is a one-step problem.
   Step 1: 2.2 lb:1 kg::14 lb:x kg   PROOF: $1 \times 14 = 14$
   　　　　2.2x = 14   　　　　$2.2 \times 6.36 = 13.99$ or 14
   　　　　x = 6.36 kg

   b. 12.2 oz = approximately 6 kg
   This is a two-step problem.
   Step 1: oz to lb
   　　　　16 oz:1 lb::2 oz:x lb   PROOF: $16 \times 0.12 = 1.92$
   　　　　16x = 2   　　　　$1 \times 2 = 2$
   　　　　x = ⅛ or .12 lb   Total weight: 12.12 lb

   Step 2: lb to kg
   　　　　2.2 lb:1 kg::12.12:x kg   PROOF: $1 \times 12.12 = 12.12$
   　　　　2.2x = 12.12   　　　　$5.5 \times 2.2 = 12.1$
   　　　　x = 5.5 kg

   c. 7 lb, 6 oz = approximately 3.5 kg
   Step 1: oz to lb
   　　　　16 oz:1 lb::6 oz:x PROOF: $1 \times 6 = 6$
   　　　　16x = 6   　　　　$16 \times 0.37 = 5.92$ or 6
   　　　　x = 0.37 lb   Total weight: 7.37 lb

   Step 2: lb to kg

Know	**Want to know**

   　　　　2.2 lb:1 kg::7.37 lb:x kg   PROOF: $1 \times 7.37 = 7.37$
   　　　　2.2x = 7.37   　　　　$2.2 \times 3.35 = 7.37$
   　　　　x = 3.35 kg

d. 15 lb, 8 oz = approximately 7.5 kg

Step 1: oz to lb

Know	**Want to know**

16 oz:1 lb::8 oz:x lb   PROOF: $16 \times .5 = 8$

$16x = 8$ $1 \times 8 = 8$

$x = 0.5$ lb   Total weight: 15.5 lb

Step 2: lb to kg

Know	**Want to know**

2.2 lb:1 kg::15.5 lb:x kg   PROOF: $2.2 \times 7 = 15.4$

$2.2x = 15.5$ $1 \times 15.5 = 15.5$

$x = 7.0$ kg

2. a. $150 \times 3 = 450$ mg
   b. $200 \times 4 = 800$ mg
   c. $50 \times 3 = 150$ mg
   d. $75 \times 2 = 150$ mg

3. a.
Know	**Want to know**

10 mg:1 kg::x mg:5 kg   PROOF: $10 \times 5 = 50$

$x = 10 \times 5$ or 50 mg $1 \times 50 = 50$

b.
Know	**Want to know**

Step 1: 5 mg:1 kg::x mg:7.3 kg   PROOF: $5 \times 7.3 = 36.5$

$x = 5 \times 7.3$ or 36.5 mg $1 \times 36.5 = 36.5$

Know	**Want to know**

Step 2: 8 mg:1 kg::x mg:7.3 kg   PROOF: $8 \times 7.3 = 58.4$

$x = 8 \times 7.3$ or 58.4 mg $1 \times 58.4 = 58.4$

c. 8 lb = approximately 4 kg

   Step 1: lb to kg

        Know   **Want to know**

        2.2 lb:1 kg::8 lb:x kg   PROOF: $2.2 \times 3.63 = 7.98$

        $2.2x = 8$ $1 \times 8 = 8$

        $x = 3.63$ kg   (Estimate was 4 kg.)

        Know   **Want to know**

   Step 2: 6 mg:1 kg::x mg:3.63 kg   PROOF: $1 \times 21.78 = 21.78$

        $x = 21.78$ mg $6 \times 3.63 = 21.78$

        Know   **Want to know**

   Step 3: 8 mg:1 kg::x mg:3.63 kg   PROOF: $1 \times 29.04 = 29.04$

        $x = 29.04$ mg $8 \times 3.63 = 29.04$

        Answer range is 21.78 mg to 29.04 mg.

d. Estimate kg.

        Know   **Want to know**

   Step 1: 16 oz:1 lb::8 oz:x lb   PROOF: $16 \times 0.5 = 8.0$

        $16x = 8$ $1 \times 8 = 8$

        $x = 0.5$ lb

        Know   **Want to know**

   Step 2: 2.2 lb:1 kg::5.5 lb:x kg   PROOF: $1 \times 5.5 = 5.5$

        $2.2x = 5.5$ $2.2 \times 2.5 = 5.5$

        $x = 2.5$ kg (Estimate was 2.5 kg.)

        Know   **Want to know**

   Step 3: 3 mg:1 kg::x mg:2.5 kg   PROOF: $3 \times 2.5 = 7.5$

        $x = 7.5$ kg $1 \times 7.5 = 7.5$

        Know   **Want to know**

        6 mg:1 kg::x mg:2.5 kg   PROOF: $6 \times 2.5 = 15$

        $x = 15.0$ mg $1 \times 15 = 15$

        Answer range is 7.5 to 15 mg.

1. *mg/kg method*

   weight in kg: 7 lb, 2 oz = approximately 3.5 kg

   Know   **Want to know**

   16 oz:1 lb::2 oz:x lb   PROOF: $1 \times 2 = 2$

   $$\frac{16x}{x} = \frac{2}{16} = \frac{1}{8} = 0.125 \text{ lb}$$ $16 \times 0.25 = 2$

   Know   **Want to know**

   2.2 lb:1 kg::7.125 lb:x kg   PROOF: $2.2 \times 3.23 = 7.106$

   $2.2x = 7.125$ $1 \times 7.125 = 7.125$

   $x = 3.23$ kg baby weight

   safe ranges:

   Know   **Want to know**

   3 mg:1 kg::x mg:3.23 kg   PROOF: $3 \times 3.23 = 9.69$

   $x = 9.69$ mg low safe dose for 24 hours $1 \times 9.69 = 9.69$

   Know   **Want to know**

   6 mg:1 kg::x mg:3.23 kg   PROOF: $6 \times 3.23 = 19.38$

   $x = 19.38$ mg maximum safe dose for 24 hours $1 \times 19.38 = 19.38$

   Doctor ordered 10 mg $\times$ 4 or 40 mg total.
   Safe range is 9.69 mg to 19.38 mg for this baby.
   Unsafe order. Hold and clarify promptly.

2. *BSA method*

   $$\frac{0.52}{1.7} \times 60 = 18 \text{ mg safe individual dose for this child}$$

   Have   **Want to know**

   80 mg:2 ml::18 mg:x ml   PROOF: $80 \times 0.45 = 36$

   $80x = 36$ $2 \times 18 = 36$

   $x = 0.45$ ml

3. *BSA method*

$$\frac{0.6}{1.7} \times 60 = 21 \text{ mg safe individual dose for this child}$$

Know   **Want to know**

4 mg:1 kg::x mg:13.6 kg   PROOF: $1 \times 54.4 = 54.4$
$x = 4 \times 13.6$ or 54.4 mg/24 hours order $4 \times 13.6 = 54.4$

54.5 mg:3 dose::x mg:1 dose   PROOF: $1 \times 54.5 = 54.5$
$3x = 54.5$ $3 \times 18.1 = 54.3$
$x = 18.1$ mg ordered per dose

21 mg is safe individual dose (BSA method).
18.1 mg per dose is ordered for this baby.
Safe order.

Have   **Want to know**

10 mg:1 ml::18.1 mg:x ml   PROOF: $10 \times 1.8 = 18$
$10x = 18.1$ $1 \times 18.1 = 18.1$
$x = 1.8$ ml

4. *mg/kg method*
   estimated kg = 2.5

Know   **Want to know**

16 oz:1 lb::10 oz:x lb   PROOF: $16 \times 0.62 = 9.9$
$16x = 10$ $1 \times 10 = 10$
$x = 0.62$
Baby weighs 5.62 lb.

Know   **Want to know**

2.2 lb:1 kg::5.62 lb:x kg   PROOF: $2.2 \times 2.55 = 5.619$
$2.2x = 5.62$ $1 \times 5.62 = 5.62$
$x = 2.55$ kg
Baby weighs 2.55 kg.

Know   **Want to know**

50 mg:1 kg::x mg:2.55 kg   PROOF: $50 \times 2.55 = 127.5$
$50x = 2.55$ $1 \times 127.5 = 127.5$
$x = 127.5$ mg safe 24-hour dosage

24 hr MD order is 50×3 or 150 mg.
Safe limit for 24 hr (mg/kg method) is 127.5 mg.
Unsafe order. Hold and clarify promptly.

5. *mg/kg method*
   estimated weight $= 4.5$ kg

   Know   **Want to know**

   16 oz:1 lb::2 oz:x lb   PROOF: $16 \times 0.125 = 2$

   $16x = 2$ $1 \times 2 = 2$

   $x = 0.125$ lb   Baby weighs 9.125 lb.

   Know   **Want to know**

   2.2 lb:1 kg::9.125:x lb   PROOF: $2.2 \times 4.14 = 9.108$

   $2.2x = 9.125$ $1 \times 9.125 = 9.125$

   $x = 4.14$ kg

   Know   **Want to know**

   20 mg:1 kg::x mg:4.14 kg   PROOF: $20 \times 4.14 = 82.8$

   $x = 20 \times 4.14$ or 82.8 mg q.12h. $1 \times 82.8 = 82.8$

   24 hr order is 40 mg $\times$ 2 or 80 mg.
   Safe 24 hr dosage by mg/kg method is 82.8 mg $\times$ 2 or 165.6 mg.
   Safe order.

   Have   **Want to know**

   300 mg:1 ml::40 mg:x ml   PROOF: $300 \times 0.13 = 39$

   $300x = 40$ $1 \times 40 = 40$

   $x = 0.13$ ml

11D Answer sheet

1. *mg/kg method*

    30 lb = approximately 15 kg

    Know   **Want to know**

    2.2 lb:1 kg::30 lb:x kg   PROOF: $1 \times 30 = 30$
    $2.2x = 30$ $2.3 \times 13.6 = 29.92$ or 30
    $x = 13.6$ kg

    Know   **Want to know**

    5 mg:1 kg::x mg:13.6 kg   PROOF: $5 \times 13.6 = 68$
    $x = 13.6 \times 5$ or 68.0 mg $1 \times 68 = 68$

    24 hr order = $30 \times 3 = 90$ mg
    Safe 24 hr dose = 68 mg
    Hold and clarify stat.

2. *mg/kg method*

    12 lb = approximately 6 kg

    Know   **Want to know**

    16 oz:1 lb::4 oz:x lb   PROOF: $16 \times .25 = 4$
    $16x = 4$ $1 \times 4 = 4$
    $x = 0.25$ lb   Baby weighs 12.25 lb.

    Know   **Want to know**

    2.2 lb:1 kg::12.25:x kg   PROOF: $2.2 \times 5.56 = 12.232$
    $2.2x = 12.25$ $1 \times 12.25 = 12.25$
    $x = 5.56$ kg

    Know   **Want to know**

    100 mg:1 kg::x mg:5.56 kg   PROOF: $1 \times 556 = 556$
    $x = 556$ mg low safe 24 hr dose $100 \times 5.56 = 556$

    200 mg:1 kg::x mg:5.56 kg   PROOF: $1 \times 1112 = 1112$
    $x = 1112$ mg maximum safe dose 24 hr $200 \times 5.56 = 1112$

    Doctor ordered 800 mg for 24 hr.
    Safe order.

    Know   **Want to know**

    125 mg:5 ml::200 mg:x ml   PROOF: $5 \times 200 = 1000$
    $125x = 1000$ $125 \times 8 = 1000$
    $x = 8$ ml

3. $\dfrac{20 \text{ lb}}{150} \times 8 = \dfrac{16}{15} = 1.06 \text{ ml}$

4. $\dfrac{30 \text{ lb}}{150} \times 5 = \dfrac{5}{5} = 1 \text{ mg}$

   Have   **Want to know**

   10 mg : 2 ml : : 1 mg : x ml   PROOF: $2 \times 1 = 2$

   $10x = 2$ $10 \times 0.2 = 2.0$

   $x = 0.2 \text{ ml}$

5. $\dfrac{0.84}{1.7} \times 30 = \dfrac{25.2}{1.7} = 14.8 \text{ mg}$

   10 mg h.s. is a safe dose.

Section 11 CHILDREN'S DOSAGES QUIZ

Solve the following problems by using the *mg/kg* rules*:

1. The doctor ordered tetracycline 200 mg IV b.i.d. for a child who weighs 45 lb. Safe range is 10 to 20 mg/kg/day in two divided doses. On hand are 250 mg vials of sterile tetracycline hydrochloride that are to be reconstituted initially with 5 ml of sterile water for injection. What is safe dosage range for this child? Is the order safe? If so, how many ml will you withdraw from the vial?

2. The doctor ordered Keflin 250 mg IM q.6h. for a child who weighs 20 lb, 4 oz. Safe range for children is 80 to 160 mg/kg. What is the safe dosage range for this child? Is the order safe? If so, how many ml will you withdraw from the vial? On hand is a 1 g vial that can be reconstituted with 4 ml for IM use.

3. The doctor ordered Lasix 20 mg p.o. stat for a child. The safe dosage for initial therapy is 2 mg/kg. The child weighed 25 lb today. What is the safe dosage for this child's weight? Is the order safe? If so, how many ml will you give? On hand is Lasix Oral Solution 10 mg/ml.

*Calculate kg to hundredths.

Solve the following problems by using Clark's rule:

4. Adult dose of ampicillin is 600,000 U. How much would a child weighing 90 lb receive? Available is ampicillin 300,000 U/ml. How many ml will you give?

5. Adult dose of penicillin is 600,000 units. How much would a 75 lb child receive? Available is penicillin 600,000 U/2 ml. How many ml will you give?

6. The average adult dose of ASA is 650 mg. A child weighing 40 lb would require how many mg? The bottle of chewable baby aspirin reads: "Each tablet contains gr 1¼." How many tablets will you give? Use BSA method.

Solve the following pediatric problems:

7. Doctor ordered Mintezol 25 mg/kg of body weight. If the child weighs 20 kg, how many mg will you give? The bottle reads: "Each 5 ml contains 250 mg." How many ml will you give?

8. Doctor ordered gr iii Liquiprin. Bottle contains 60 mg per 1.25 ml. The dropper measures 2.5 ml. How many ml will you give?

9. On hand is a pediatric oral suspension of Veetids '250' (penicillin-V potassium). The bottle contains 10 g. Directions read: ''Add 117 ml water to prepare 200 ml oral solution.'' Doctor ordered 1 tsp. q.i.d. × 10 days. How many mg will each tsp. contain?

10. Average dose of Kantrex (kanamycin sulfate) daily is 750 to 1000 mg. Directions read: ''15 mg/kg in divided doses not to exceed 1.5 g in 1 day.'' The baby weighs 8 lb. How many mg of Kantrex should the baby receive?

Section 11 Children's dosages quiz answer sheet _____

1. Safe range is 204.5 to 409 mg daily.
   Safe order; withdraw 4 ml.

2. Safe dosage range is 736 mg to 1472 mg. Withdraw 1 ml from vial for 250 mg per dose.

3. Safe dosage is 22.72 mg. Order is safe at 20 mg. Give 2 ml p.o. stat.

4. 360,000 units. Give 1.2 ml IM.

5. 300,000 units. Give 1 ml IM.

6. 267 mg. Give 3½ tablets.

7. 500 mg. Give 10 ml or 2 tsp.

8. Measure 3.75 ml. Measure one full dropper with 2.5 ml and then measure to 1.25 ml calibration on the dropper again to complete the dose.

9. Each tsp. will contain 250 mg.

10. 54 mg

Comprehensive quiz

Show work, label answers, and prove:

1. Doctor has ordered elix. of phenobarbital 0.5 g p.o. a.c. t.i.d. The label reads "elix. of phenobarb. 250 mg/ml." How many ml for each dose? How many per day?

2. Doctor orders quinidine 200 mg IM. On hand is a vial labeled "quinidine 0.1 g/3 ml." How many ml will you give?

3. Doctor orders 500 mg of Diuril. On hand are 0.25 g tablets. How many tablets?

4. You are to give atropine gr $^1/_{200}$. On hand is a vial labeled "gr $^1/_{150}$ in 0.5 cc." How many ml will you give?

5. You are to give 200,000 units of penicillin. On hand is a multiple-dose vial labeled "1,000,000 U in 10 cc." How many ml will you give?

6. A patient is to receive 500 ml of NS intravenously in 8 hr. How many ml/hr should the patient receive?

7. The above as an IV dose should be infused at _____ gtt/min. Drop factor is 15.

8. The patient is to receive 1000 ml of D5W in 8 hr. How many ml/hr will that be?

9. An IV fluid is being infused at a rate of 100 ml/hr. This should run at _____ gtt/min. Drop factor is 10 gtt/ml.

10. Doctor ordered penicillin 300,000 units. On hand is a penicillin 5 ml vial stating: "Add 5 ml sterile H_2O to make penicillin 600,000 U/2 ml." How many ml will you give?

11. You are to give penicillin 1.3 million units stat. On hand is a vial labeled "10,000,000 units in 10 ml." You will give _____ ml.

12. Ordered: penicillin 600,000 units IM q.8h. Available: penicillin 2,000,000 units per 5 ml. You will give _____ ml every 8 hr.

13. Ordered is codeine gr ¹/₆. On hand is gr ¹/₄ per ml. How many ml will you give?

14. On hand: codeine (tablets) gr ¹/₂ p.o. Ordered: 60 mg. How many tablets will you give?

15. Ordered: digoxin 0.125 mg. On hand is an ampule labeled "digoxin 0.25 mg/ml." How many ml will you give?

16. Doctor ordered 24 units of U 100 every AM ¹/₂ hr a.c. regular insulin. You are out of insulin syringes. How many ml will you give in a tuberculin syringe?

17. Ordered is atropine gr $^1/_{200}$. On hand is atropine gr $^1/_{150}$ per 0.5 cc. How many minims will you give?

18. Ordered: heparin sodium 5000 U stat. On hand you have a vial labeled "heparin sodium 20,000 U per ml." How many ml will you give (nearest hundredth)?

19. Ordered: 75 mg meperidine and vistaril 25 mg on call to the O.R. Have: demerol 100 mg/ml in a prefilled tube and a 2 ml vial of vistaril containing 100 mg. How many total ml will you prepare? (Round off to tenths.)

20. Ordered: atropine sulfate gr $^1/_{150}$. The pharmacist has sent atropine sulfate 0.43 mg/0.5 ml. How many ml will you give?

21. Prepare a normal saline solution (0.9%) as a gargle for a sore throat. You will use _____ tsp. of table salt per pint of water.

22. Doctor ordered aminophylline suppository 0.5 g. On hand you have aminophylline suppository gr $vii\overline{ss}$. How many will you give?

23. Doctor ordered ASA 0.9 g. The tablets available are labeled "325 mg." How many tablets will you give?

24. Your weight is 55 kg. This is equivalent to how many lb? (Estimate first.)

25. Doctor ordered tetracycline 100 mg IV b.i.d. for a child who weighs 15 lb, 8 oz. Safe range is 10 to 20 mg/kg/day in two divided doses. On hand are 250 mg vials of sterile tetracycline hydrochloride that are to be reconstituted initially with 5 ml of sterile water for injection. What is the safe dosage range for this child? Is the order safe? If so, how many ml will you withdraw from the vial?

26. Ordered: thyroid tablets 120 mg daily A.M. On hand are tablets labeled "thyroid gr i." How many tablets or part of a tablet will you give?

27. Doctor ordered ℥ ss of elixer of terpin hydrate with codeine. How many ml will you give? How many teaspoons is this?

28. Convert 101° F to C (Celsius). See Appendix C.

Comprehensive quiz answer sheet

1. 2 ml dose and 6 ml per day
2. 6 ml
3. 2 tablets
4. 0.4 ml
5. 2 ml
6. 63 ml/hr
7. 16 gtt/min
8. 125 ml/hr
9. 17 gtt/min
10. 1 ml
11. 1.3 ml
12. 1.5 ml
13. 0.7 ml
14. 2 tablets
15. 0.5 ml
16. 0.24 ml
17. 6 minims
18. 0.25 ml
19. 1.3 ml
20. 0.5 ml
21. 1 tsp.
22. 1 suppository
23. 3 tablets
24. 121 lb
25. 70 to 141 mg; unsafe
26. 2 tablets
27. 15 ml or 3 tsp.
28. 38.3° C

APPENDIX A

Abbreviations for medications

ā or a.	before	H.	hypodermically
aa, āa, or āa	of each	h. or hr	hour
a.c.	before meals	h.s.	hour of sleep (bedtime)
ad lib	as desired, freely		
alt. h.	alternate hours	IM	intramuscular(ly)
AM	in the morning, before noon	inj.	injection
		IV	intravenous(ly)
aq.	water	kg	kilogram
b.i.d.	twice a day	L	liter
b.i.n.	twice a night	lb	pound
C	gallon, Celsius	liq.	liquid
c̄	with	M, m	meter
cap. or caps.	capsule	ɱ, ɱ, or m.	minim
cc	cubic centimeter	m̶	mix
comp.	compound	mcg	microgram (μg preferable)
d.	day; right (properly only *dexter*, *dextra*)		
		mEq	milliequivalent
		mg	milligram
dil.	dilute	μg	microgram
dist.	distilled	mixt.	mixture
dr	dram	ml	milliliter
elix.	elixir	n.	night
et	and	no.	number
ext.	external, extract	noct.	night
F	Fahrenheit	non rep.	do not repeat
fl. or fld.	fluid	O.	pint
g	gram	o.	every; eye
gr	grain	o.d.	every day
gtt	drop	O.D.	right eye

o.h., omn. hor.	every hour	q.4h.	every 4 hours
o.s.	left eye	q.6h.	every 6 hours
o.n.	every night	q.8h.	every 8 hours
o.u.	in each eye	q.12h.	every 12 hours
oz	ounce	q.s.	as much as needed
$\overline{p}$ or p.	after; per	qt	quart
p̱	per	rep.	repeat
p.c.	after meals	$\overline{s}$	without
p.o., per os	by mouth	$\overline{ss}$ or ss	half
PM	afternoon; evening	SC	subcutaneously
p.r.n.	as needed, when necessary, according to circumstances	sol. or soln.	solution
		s.o.s.	if needed
		SQ/sub $\overline{q}$	subcutaneous
pt	pint	stat.	immediately, at once
pulv.	powder	tab.	tablet
q.	each, every	tbs.	tablespoon
q.d.	every day	t.i.d.	three times a day
q.h.	every hour	tinct. or tr.	tincture
q.i.d.	four times a day	tsp.	teaspoon
q.1h.	every hour	U	unit
q.2h.	every 2 hours	μg	microgram
q.3h.	every 3 hours		

Drug classifications

Drugs are classified according to their action or use:

1. Antiseptics and disinfectants
   a. Halogens
   b. Heavy metals
   c. Oxidizing agents
   d. Phenol group
   e. Various dyes
   f. Miscellaneous (alcohol, benzyl benzoate lotion, formaldehyde)
2. Anti-infectives
   a. Antibiotics
   b. Specific anti-infectives (antiviral and antibacterial)
3. Biologicals
   a. Allergens
   b. Serums
   c. Testing materials
   d. Toxoids
   e. Vaccines
4. Drugs affecting autonomic nervous system
   a. Sympathomimetics (sympathetic stimulants)
   b. Cholinergic drugs
   c. Anticholinergic drugs (e.g., atropine)
5. Drugs affecting central nervous system
   a. Stimulants
   b. Antidepressants
   c. Depressants
      (1) Intoxicants (e.g., alcohol)
      (2) Analgesics
         (a) Narcotic antagonists
         (b) Drugs used for potentiating analgesia
         (c) Antipyretics
      (3) Barbiturates and sedatives
      (4) Antispasmodics
         (a) Anticonvulsants
         (b) Muscle relaxants

(5) Psychotherapeutic agents
   (a) Tranquilizers
   (b) Antidepressants
(6) General and local anesthetics

6. Antihistamines
7. Histamines
8. Drugs affecting circulatory system
   a. Digitalis and related heart drugs
   b. Diuretics
   c. Antiarrhythmics
   d. Antihypertensives
   e. Calcium ion blockers
   f. Anticoagulants
   g. Hematinics
   h. Vasodilators
9. Drugs acting on gastrointestinal system
   a. Antacids
   b. Emetics
   c. Antiemetics
   d. Antiseptics
   e. Adsorbents, antidiarrheals
   f. Cathartics
   g. Stool softeners
10. Drugs acting on endocrine system
   a. Hormones
11. Drugs affecting respiratory system
   a. Stimulants
   b. Bronchodilators
   c. Cough medications
12. Drugs acting on urinary system
   a. Acidifiers, alkalinizers
   b. Antiseptics
   c. Diuretics
13. Drugs affecting skeletal system
   a. Anti-inflammatory agents
   b. Muscle relaxants
14. Miscellaneous
   a. Drugs used for alcoholism
   b. Vitamins/minerals
   c. Enzymes

APPENDIX C

Temperature conversion

To convert Fahrenheit to Celsius:

1. Subtract 32
2. Multiply by 5
3. Divide by 9

EXAMPLE: Change 102° F to Celsius.

1.
```
   102
  − 32
   70
```

2.
```
   ×5
   350
```

3.
```
      38.8° C
   9)350.
      27
      80
      72
       8
```

To convert Celsius to Fahrenheit:

1. Multiply by 9
2. Divide by 5
3. Add 32

EXAMPLE: Change 36° C to Fahrenheit.

1.
```
   36
   ×9
   324
```

2.
```
      64.8
   5)324.0
      30
      24
      20
       4
       4 0
```

3.
```
   64.8
   32.0
   96.8° F
```